Nutritional Supplements

for the Veterinary Practice

A Pocket Guide

Shawn Messonnier, DVM

Edited by Nancy Scanlan, DVM, MSFP, CVA

AAHA
press

This book is dedicated to the two most important
people in my life: Sandy and Erica.

American Animal Hospital Association Press
12575 West Bayaud Avenue
Lakewood, Colorado 80228

Acquisitions Editor: Bess Maher
Developmental/Medical Editor: Stacey Oke

Book design: Laura Hartgerink/Signify, LLC
Cover images: herbal silhouettes © istockphoto/Helga Jaunegg; cat
silhouette © istockphoto/pixitive; dog silhouette © istockphoto/Igor
Diurovic.

ISBN 978-1-58326-174-3
Cataloging-in-Publication Data is available from the Library of Congress.

Printed in Canada
12 13 14 / 10 9 8 7 6 5 4 3 2 1

CONTENTS

PREFACE

The use of nutritional and herbal supplements continues to grow each year. Most (if not all) veterinarians currently recommend some type of nutritional supplementation for their patients such as fish oil, glucosamine, and antioxidants. Unfortunately, many pet owners continue to use supplements (for themselves as well as their pets) with no medical supervision. This can result in inadequate dosing, misdiagnosis because the pet has potentially never been examined by a veterinarian, toxicity from the supplement, interactions with other supplements or medications prescribed by the veterinarian or given to the pet by the owner, and/or the development of side effects causing patient morbidity and possibly mortality. This book, *Nutritional Supplements for the Veterinary Practice: A Pocket Guide*, was written to address these concerns. For the first time, veterinarians and veterinary technical and support staff have at their disposal information on natural supplements presented in a concise and easy-to-use fashion. Typical of a true handbook, *Nutritional Supplements for the Veterinary Practice: A Pocket Guide* is not meant to be a thorough, in-depth discussion of everything that is known about natural supplements. Instead, this handbook is meant to be a user-friendly resource that can help provide essential and accurate information as quickly as possible for the busy practitioner and office staff, as well as resources for readers who wish to obtain additional information.

Although there is an ever-increasing amount of accurate information on the topic of natural supplements in people, there is still scant literature involving well-researched studies on the use of many of the commercially available natural supplements in pets. Much of the information in the veterinary literature is based on case reports and anecdotal/common usage of supplements, and is extrapolated from the human literature. Nonetheless, veterinarians are sharing information about potentially efficacious doses of supplements that seem to be helping their patients. Still, natural therapies can be used safely despite the deficiencies in our knowledge base (because of the lack of well-designed, controlled clinical studies). With more experience and (hopefully) more research, our knowledge base will continue to grow. Until then, *Nutritional Supplements for the Veterinary Practice: A Pocket Guide* will help guide you in your endeavors to use natural therapies.

Several copies of this handbook might benefit your veterinary hospital. One can serve as a reference in the library, one or more copies can serve as working copies, and another can be kept in the examination rooms or the pharmacy to facilitate rapid dosing information. Finally, one copy can be placed in the waiting room to encourage pet owners to feel comfortable discussing the topic of natural therapies with either the veterinarians or veterinary technical staff. This will instill confidence in the pet owners that the staff is able to accurately recommend appropriate supplements for their pets.

While writing this book, I attempted to be as accurate as possible and provide as many references as possible regarding the use of nutritional supplements in pets. I believe that *Nutritional Supplements for the Veterinary Practice: A Pocket Guide* will serve the needs of the veterinary community and will be frequently used in clinical practice. My hope is that this book will serve as a starting point for future books on the topic and will encourage more research so that the "science" part of natural medicine will grow with the "art" of natural medicine. I welcome hearing from readers of any recommendations or suggestions for future editions. You can contact me at shawnvet@sbcglobal.net.

Shawn Messonnier, DVM
February 2012

ACKNOWLEDGMENTS

I would like to thank the wonderful people at AAHA Press, especially my editor Bess Maher. Thank you for believing in this project and making it come to life. I'm looking forward to working with you on many more such projects in the future. I would like to thank my colleague Dr. Nancy Scanlan for her valuable review of the manuscript at various stages and her assistance in providing additional references for the supplements included in this book, all my mentors in the world of naturopathic medicine and naturopathic veterinary medicine, my wonderful staff at Paws & Claws Animal Hospital for running a tight ship when I'm busy writing and am not able to be at the office, and the wonderful clients who seek natural healing for their pets at my hospital. Your dedication to your pets is amazing. Finally, I would like to thank God for giving me the wonderful opportunity to discover the natural healing ability he put in all of us.

INTRODUCTION

What Is a Nutritional Supplement?

The term "nutritional supplement" refers to any product taken by mouth that contains one or more "dietary ingredients" intended to supplement the diet. These dietary ingredients can include vitamins; minerals; herbs or other botanicals (also referred to as natural products); amino acids; substances such as enzymes, organ tissues, glandulars, and metabolites; and extracts or concentrates. Nutritional supplements are available in many forms, such as tablets, capsules, softgels, gelcaps, liquids, and powders. They are also available as tasty treats (e.g., dog biscuits and chews).[1] Nutritional supplements, also referred to as dietary supplements or food supplements, are considered complementary and alternative medicine (CAM), which is one of many medical healthcare products or techniques that can be used either instead of or in conjunction with conventional medical practices.[2] Other examples of CAM are acupuncture and chiropractic.

In veterinary medicine, just as in human medicine, the use of nutritional supplements has become extremely popular over the past few decades. Surveys show that more than 20% of all dog owners and 15% of cat owners currently offer some type of nutritional supplement to their pets. The most popular nutritional supplements for pets are those for joints, general multivitamins, skin/coat, and digestive health. By 2015, annual U.S. sales of pet nutritional supplements are expected to exceed $2 billion, of which products for dogs and cats are anticipated to account for almost 60% of the market.[3] As described below and mentioned earlier in the Preface, not all supplements are created equal. For that reason, owners should be encouraged to use nutritional supplements under the advice and guidance of a veterinarian.

Natural Versus Synthetic

The term "natural" is used extensively when referring to nonconventional medical therapies such as nutritional supplements. Natural therapies are also referred to as "holistic," "complementary," and "alternative" therapies. To my knowledge there is no one agreed-upon definition of the term "natural." In general, the term "natural" is meant to imply "from nature" as opposed to "man-made or chemically derived." For example, consider white willow bark and its conventional medical derivative, acetylsalicylic acid (aspirin). White willow bark contains salicin plus numerous other ingredients, but salicin is the active ingredient responsible for the pharmacologic properties of white willow bark. History records Hippocrates prescribing the leaves and bark of the white willow tree to relieve pain and fever in 400 BC. In 1897, the Bayer Company extracted salicin from white willow bark and chemically modified it to form acetylsalicylic acid. The main difference between the salicin contained in white willow bark and acetylsalicylic acid contained in aspirin is one acetyl group (a small organic moiety with a carbon molecule double bonded to an oxygen and single bonded to another carbon with three hydrogens). This small modification resulted in a product (aspirin) that confers antithrombotic properties (prevents the formation of blood clots), which is not a property of white willow bark. A naturopathic practitioner who wants the pharmacologic benefits of aspirin, such as the anti-inflammatory effects, would likely prescribe the "natural" form by prescribing the herb white willow bark to his or her patients, whereas a conventional doctor would prescribe the chemically made conventional drug acetylsalicylic acid (aspirin).

This example may make the distinction between natural and man-made relatively straightforward, but in reality things are not nearly so cut and dry, and sometimes the lines between the two types of products are blurred. For example, consider the herb milk thistle. The active ingredient in milk thistle is silymarin. There are currently several commercially available silymarin supplements for pets. These supplements might be considered "natural" to some consumers, but for them to be considered truly "natural," a practitioner would have to prescribe the raw herb milk thistle rather than a silymarin supplement that is made from chemically extracting the silymarin from the raw herb. Unless the practitioner is well versed in herbal medicine, it is unlikely that he or she would prescribe the raw herb. Instead, he or she would likely recommend one of the several currently marketed silymarin supplements. The problem is that silymarin supplements often contain only one ingredient (silymarin). In contrast, the raw herb milk thistle contains many other ingredients that might be beneficial. Some of the commercially available silymarin supplements might also contain other ingredients, such as artificial dyes or flavors, which may or may not be "natural." Thus, doctors and pet owners who want to use more "natural" products than chemically derived or synthetic products often prefer supplements over conventional medications. In reality, however, most of our supplements (except for raw herbs) are not as "natural" as we might like or expect.

Art Versus Science

Veterinary practitioners are well versed in the scientific aspects of medicine, so it is easy to forget that medicine is also an art. As you read this book, it will become apparent that well-designed controlled research studies are often lacking for many of the supplements that are discussed, particularly in veterinary medicine. This is where the "art" part of medicine comes into play. By understanding the biochemistry of a particular supplement and seeing how it might be used in people (where there are more well-designed controlled studies), veterinarians can extrapolate and identify medical conditions that might be amenable to supplementation with a particular product or ingredient.

Not Perfect, but the Science Is There

One of the most common complaints from those who express opposition to the use of natural therapies such as nutritional supplements is the lack of credible scientific evidence "proving" the efficacy of such therapies. This complaint is valid at times; however, this lack of evidence should not preclude the use of natural therapies that may help veterinary patients.

While researching for *Nutritional Supplements for the Veterinary Practice: A Pocket Guide,* several issues regarding the amount of scientific evidence quickly became apparent. First, there are many studies in the human medical literature showing the effectiveness of natural therapies, including nutritional supplements. Second, there is a relative deficiency of the same type and quality of evidence in the veterinary medical literature. Third, as a result of this deficiency in the veterinary medical literature, recommendations regarding the use of natural therapies, including nutritional supplements, in pets must be based on the available scientific evidence, including extrapolation from the human medical literature as well as case reports, clinical experience, historical usage, and anecdotal usage of these therapies. This approach is problematic at times, and common sense must be used to offer sound guidelines based on whatever credible scientific evidence exists in order to be able to help our veterinary patients. Fourth, even the credible scientific evidence in the human medical literature is not perfect. For example, in researching various herbs it became apparent that there were (at times) conflicting studies based on the form of herb used as well as the dose used. It is not always easy to extrapolate how various forms and doses of a particular nutritional supplement or ingredient in a nutritional supplement will affect a patient. In these cases, common sense coupled with a scientific understanding of the potential actions and side effects of the herb (or other ingredient) is needed to attempt to apply research findings to clinical practice. Fifth, and finally, there are side effects reported with various supplements that may not really exist. For example, isolated case reports of certain herbs interfering with blood clotting are replete with improperly recorded information, such as concurrent herb or medication usage, the dose of the herb used in the supplement taken by the patient, and the part of the herb used in the supplement (not all parts of the herb are equally effective or equally toxic). Although a theoretical concern may exist about interactions among various supplements or medications, it is clear that because of poorly designed studies or case reports lacking important information, a definitive conclusion cannot be made. Thus, the practitioner is left to decide for him- or herself how to proceed.

Our current knowledge of nutritional supplements remains fairly limited. Future studies (which require funding) will likely alter our current recommendations. Despite these deficiencies, there are clear indications and safety issues that are adequately addressed in the medical literature to guide our prescribing of natural therapies. With these deficiencies in mind, *Nutritional Supplements for the Veterinary Practice: A Pocket Guide* contains up-to-date scientific information and can therefore guide practitioners as they seek to help their patients with nutritional supplements.

"Natural" Is Not Necessarily "Safe"

One of the most common misconceptions about "natural" therapies is that all natural therapies are safe. Somehow we have equated "natural" with "safe." When properly used, natural therapies tend to have a greater safety profile than most conventional medications do. It is equally true, however, that natural therapies can and do cause problems in patients. As an example, improperly diluted tea tree oil can be toxic and even fatal to dogs and cats. Nutritional supplements, such as herbs, often have numerous ingredients and therefore numerous pharmacological actions. Not all of these actions are known or understood. Throughout this book, I have attempted to point out safety issues most likely to be of concern to the veterinarian and veterinary support staff. Potential side effects caused by the supplement and interactions with other medications or supplements that may adversely affect the patient are important to appreciate and relay to clients.

References

1. U.S. Department of Health and Human Services United States Food and Drug Administration. Overview of Dietary Supplements. Available at: http://www.fda .gov/Food/DietarySupplements/ConsumerInformation/ucm110417.htm#what. Accessed January 15, 2012.

2. National Institutes of Health National Center for Complementary and Alternative Medicine. What is complementary and alternative medicine? Available at: http://nccam.nih.gov/health/whatiscam/. Accessed January 15, 2012.

3. Packaged Facts. Pet Supplements and Nutraceutical Treats in the U.S., 3rd edition. February 2011. Available at: https://www.packagedfacts.com/Pet -Supplements-Nutraceutical-2588715/. Accessed January 15, 2012.

HOW TO USE THIS BOOK

This book is organized alphabetically by the commonly used names of various nutritional supplements and includes 42 supplements that are most commonly used by either veterinarians or pet owners. The following categories appear in the description and discussion of each supplement: background, indications, recommended doses, side effects, contraindications, and interactions.

The "Background" section provides general information about each supplement. The information is presented in a concise manner that allows the healthcare professional to have a clear (but brief) understanding of the biochemistry of the supplement (i.e., how the supplement is thought to work).

The "Indications" section lists one or more *suggested* uses for each supplement for humans, dogs, and cats. These uses are based on research and/or clinical experience. Information on the use of each nutritional supplement is also provided for humans because most of the research on nutritional supplements has been performed in humans. In addition, there may be a use for a particular supplement in people that does not occur in pets (such as AIDS); however, similar conditions in pets (such as FIV) could potentially benefit from the supplement.

The "Recommended Doses" section provides doses for humans, dogs, and cats wherever possible. This is because some doses for some supplements used in people have been established through clinical studies; however, these same supplements may not have been studied in pets. In many instances, the doses listed in this handbook for pets are those that have been reported in the literature or listed on the manufacturer-derived labels for a specific product. For all supplements, every attempt has been made to provide as much accurate information as possible regarding doses. In many cases, the clinician must use his or her own judgment in deciding the "best" dose for each particular patient. When in doubt, clinicians should start with a dose at the lower end when a dose range is given and adjust the dose based on the response of the patient. For each dose, the standard format is presented (*q* 8, 12, 24 hr, for example) or the dose/day is described if the supplement is divided into one or more doses or administered in a single dose.

Several supplements listed in *Nutritional Supplements for the Veterinary Practice: A Pocket Guide* are Western herbal supplements (i.e., supplements with a Western name rather than a Chinese name). In some cases, especially in pets, there is no agreed-upon dose for herbs. As a rule, herbalists generally recommend starting at the low end of the dose range (where available) and adjusting the dose as needed based on patient response, side effects, and/or toxicity.

It is imperative that readers appreciate that all doses are guidelines. To be safe, clinicians should prescribe herbal therapies using the following guidelines only if they are familiar with the biochemical and toxicologic properties of the herbs, because even these doses may be too high for certain pets (e.g., cats and small dogs). In addition, variability because of growing conditions of the herbs, harvesting times, and preparation methods can impact both the required and safe doses. These factors must be taken into consideration when using herbal supplements in veterinary patients.

The "Side Effects" section describes potential concerns for each supplement. The supplements included in *Nutritional Supplements for the Veterinary Practice: A Pocket Guide* are considered safe when used as recommended, so long as any potential contraindications and interactions with other medications or supplements are considered. In general, there are no studies assessing nutritional supplements in pregnant or nursing animals, and generalizations regarding the safety of these supplements in pregnant, nursing, or young animals are based on information from the human literature. Although many nutritional supplements (such as fish oil and flax) are routinely used in pregnant or nursing humans and are likely safe to use in pregnant or nursing animals, the use of herbs in these populations is more likely to be associated with possible side effects. Following label guidelines regarding the use of specific nutritional supplements in pregnant or nursing animals is helpful, but ultimately, the decision to use the supplement or herb is left to the practitioner. Initial doses should be at the low end of the recommended dose range, and patients should be carefully observed for resolution of the clinical signs and/or toxicity. **Caution is recommended when using supplements in pregnant or lactating animals and usage should be based on clinical experience with the specific supplement**.

Any known contraindication(s) associated with the administration of each supplement are described in the "Contraindications" section. Usually these contraindications apply to humans, but may be extrapolated to veterinary patients.

Finally, an "Interactions" section has been included for each nutritional supplement. Although supplements are "natural" therapies and are generally thought to be safer than conventional medical therapies, "natural" does not necessarily mean "safe." Again, the noted real or potential interactions apply to people but may be extrapolated to veterinary patients.

It is my hope that the information contained in *Nutritional Supplements for the Veterinary Practice: A Pocket Guide* will help veterinary practitioners to safely and comfortably prescribe nutritional supplements to their patients.

Nutritional
Supplements

(LIPOIC ACID, ALA)

Background

Alpha-lipoic acid (ALA) is a vitamin-like substance and enzyme cofactor that is both fat and water soluble.[1] ALA is synthesized by the body and is therefore not required in the diet, but is also found in a variety of foods such as red and organ meats and vegetables (e.g., potatoes, carrots, spinach, broccoli, beets, yams). Chemically, ALA is a carboxy acid (i.e., a weak acid containing a carbon double bonded to an oxygen molecule and the general chemical structure R-COOH) with two sulfur atoms. ALA can therefore be either oxidized or reduced, which means it can accept or donate electrons.[2] This ability to accept electrons makes ALA a potent antioxidant because it can protect cells from damage because of free radicals, which are highly reactive chemicals because of the presence of 'spare electrons.'[2] In addition, ALA chelates (binds to) heavy metals such as iron and lead.[2] Like many drugs, chemicals, and biologics, ALA occurs in nature as two "forms" called isomers, which are mirror images of the same compound. Isomers are usually referred to as either *R* and *S* or D and L. The *R*-isomer of ALA is the form synthesized naturally within the body and is the only form that functions as an enzyme cofactor.[2]

As an antioxidant, ALA not only protects cells against damaging free radicals but also preserves or recycles other antioxidants such as vitamin C, vitamin E, coenzyme Q_{10} (CoQ10), and glutathione.[2,3] ALA helps convert glucose into "energy" by acting as an enzyme cofactor (in the Krebs/citric acid cycle).[2,3] ALA is efficiently absorbed and easily crosses cell membranes, including the blood-brain barrier.[2] ALA also inhibits HIV viral replication (via inhibition of reverse transcriptase and/or increasing glutathione levels).[1] ALA regulates nuclear factor kappa B (NF-κB), which is a protein that affects the rate at which certain genes are transcribed (expressed).[2] Together, these mechanisms suggest that ALA may influence a number of processes such as inflammation, atherosclerosis, diabetes, hypertension, cancer, and acquired immunodeficiency syndrome (AIDS).[2] ALA reportedly helps protect against ocular lens damage and glaucoma,[4] diabetic neuropathy,[4] and cardiomyopathy.[5]

Indications

Suggested Uses in Humans

- Decreases blood glucose levels
- Decreases cataract formation
- Improves open-angle glaucoma
- Assists in the management of diabetic neuropathy
- Supports liver function, assists liver detoxification, and is hepato-protective (i.e., protects against chemical-, alcohol-, and Amanita mushroom poisoning–induced liver damage)
- Chelates heavy metals
- Protects against age-related cardiomyopathies
- Limits macular degeneration
- Supports cognitive function in the elderly
- Helps AIDS patients
- Supports patients with multiple sclerosis

Suggested Uses in Dogs and Cats

- Assists animals with cognitive disorders
- Helps manage diabetes mellitus and feline diabetic neuropathy
- Supports patients with peripheral neuropathy
- Limits cataracts and glaucoma
- Supports liver function in animals with chronic active hepatitis, cholangiohepatitis, and other liver diseases
- Supports patients with immune deficiency syndromes (e.g., feline immunodeficiency virus based on recommendations for treatment in people with HIV/AIDS)

Recommended Doses

Doses in people range from 100 mg to 1,800 mg *q* 24 hr. In general, the recommended dose of ALA is approximately 300–600 mg *q* 24 hr. The recommended dose for AIDS patients is 150 mg *q* 8 hr. In dogs, doses ranging from 1 mg/kg to 5 mg/kg *q* 24 hr to a maximum of 200 mg *q* 24 hr have been reported. The dose for cats is up to 25 mg/cat *q* 24 hr. It is suggested to divide the daily dose rather than giving a single dose/day.[2,4]

Side Effects

In humans, ALA is generally considered a safe supplement.[2] One notable exception is the neurologic toxicity/hepatotoxicity that can occur in cats if the daily dose exceeds 25 mg/cat/day because of ammonia accumulation. Clinical signs of ALA toxicity in cats include irritability, anorexia, ataxia, and hypersalivation.[4] Blood glucose levels may also decrease; therefore, diabetic patients taking glucose-lowering medications should be carefully monitored to prevent hypoglycemia. In people, doses of 1,200 mg *q* 24 hr for 2 years and 1,800 mg *q* 24 hr for 3 weeks produced no adverse effects.[2] Maximum safe doses in pets (other than cats) have not been established. In people, an occasional skin rash has been reported following supplementation with ALA. There has also been one report of toxicity in two dogs supplemented with ALA.[6]

Contraindications

None reported. Careful observation of diabetic patients taking glucose-lowering medications is recommended. There is (unproven) concern regarding antioxidants such as ALA possibly interfering with chemotherapy or radiation therapy, although this remains controversial.[2] Most integrative medical doctors appear comfortable with the concurrent use of antioxidants and chemotherapy/radiation therapy with careful monitoring of the patients (see Appendix 1 for a lengthier discussion of this topic).

Interactions

The antioxidant activity of ALA appears to protect people from ototoxicity and peripheral sensory neuropathy associated with the use of platinum chemotherapy medications (such as cisplatin). The use of ALA with platinum chemotherapy medications does not appear to compromise the effectiveness of the chemotherapeutics, but patients should be monitored during coadministration of ALA and platinum therapy.[2] The coadministration of ALA and aminoglycoside antibiotics (e.g., gentamicin, amikacin) may decrease renal and ototoxicity.[2] Coadministration of ALA and the antipsychotic haloperidol may reduce the haloperidol-induced glutathione depletion.[2] Coadministering ALA and angiotensin 2 receptor antagonists such as irbesartan (which are not routinely used in animals) may reduce oxidative damage in endothelial tissue, and administering ALA with insulin or oral hypoglycemic medications could result in an additive response on glucose and insulin levels.[2] Synergistic effects also likely occur with coadministration of ALA and other antioxidants (including vitamins C and E), milk thistle, acetyl-L-carnitine, coenzyme Q_{10} (CoQ10), and omega-3 fatty acids.[2]

References

1. Pizzorno J, Murray M. *Textbook of natural medicine*. 3rd ed. St. Louis (MO): Churchill Livingstone; 2006:1094–5, 1633, 1933.

2. Stargrove M, Treasure J, McKee D. *Herb, nutrient, and drug interactions: clinical implications and therapeutic strategies*. St. Louis (MO): Mosby Elsevier; 2008:718–24.

3. Broadfoot PJ, Palmquist RE, Jonston K, et al. *Integrating complementary medicine into veterinary practice*. Goldstein R, ed. Blackwell; 2008:518–32. Available at: www.mediafire.com/?2s13ctmvv7tyb2k. Accessed January 15, 2011.

4. Wynn SG, Marsden S. *Manual of natural veterinary medicine: science and tradition*. St. Louis (MO): Mosby; 2002:236, 480, 500, 510–11.

5. Li CJ, Zhang QM, Li MZ, et al. Attenuation of myocardial apoptosis by alpha-lipoic acid through suppression of mitochondrial oxidative stress to reduce diabetic cardiomyopathy. *Chin Med J* [Engl] 2009;122(21):2580–6.

6. Loftin EG, Herold LV. Therapy and outcome of suspected alpha lipoic acid toxicity in two dogs. *J Vet Emerg Crit Care* [San Antonio] 2009;19(5):501–6.

(POLLEN, PROPOLIS, ROYAL JELLY, HONEY)

Background

Bee pollen is produced from the pollination of various flowers by honeybees. Pollen comes from the male germ cell of flowering plants. Bee-related products include propolis, royal jelly, and honey. Propolis is the resinous substance collected from the leaf buds and bark of trees (especially conifer and poplar trees) used to construct the hive. Propolis possesses antimicrobial properties, which protects the hive from bacteria, viruses, and other disease-causing microorganisms. Royal jelly is a thick, milky substance produced by worker bees to feed the queen, and honey is essentially "bee vomit." Bee pollen and some bee products (excluding honey) contain sugars, proteins, essential amino acids, deoxyribonucleic acid (DNA), ribonucleic acid (RNA), flavonoids (a specific type of plant secondary metabolite), plant hormones, and vitamins and minerals, which is why they are sometimes referred to as "nature's perfect food."[1]

Bee pollen and bee-related products, especially honey, are purportedly helpful in relieving allergies.[2] The rationale is that because honey, being made from pollen, contains a number of allergenic substances, ingesting honey exposes the allergy sufferer to small doses of allergens, which may make the person more tolerant to these allergens (a theory similar to injectable antigen therapy). In the author's experience, the best response, when it occurs, is likely seen with honey produced locally, as this honey contains allergens from the environment in which the patient lives and to which the patient is most likely to develop an allergic response.

In vitro propolis has been shown to have antibacterial,[2] antifungal, antiviral, anticancer,[3] and anti-inflammatory properties.[4] Topically, propolis has shown benefit in treating wounds and burns and in healing genital herpetic lesions in people.[3] In people, bee pollen is associated with improvements in menopause symptoms, royal jelly may help with hypercholesterolemia, and propolis may be of value in patients with irritable bowel syndrome.[1]

Indications

Suggested Uses in Humans

- Improves allergies

- Enhances energy
- Alleviates menopause symptoms (pollen)
- Supports cancer patients
- Supports the immune system and fights bacterial, viral, and other infections (propolis)
- Acts as a topical anti-inflammatory agent (propolis)
- Ameliorates hypercholesterolemia (royal jelly)
- Helps manage inflammatory bowel disease

Suggested Uses in Dogs and Cats
- Improves allergies
- Helps control infectious diseases

Recommended Doses

In both people and pets, the recommended dose varies depending on the product. No standard dosing is available. Examples of approximate doses for humans are as follows: 15–45 mL (1–3 tablespoons) bee pollen *q* 24 hr, 100–500 mg propolis *q* 8 hr, 50–250 mg royal jelly *q* 12–24 hr, and 15–45 mL (1–3 tablespoons) honey *q* 24 hr.[1] In pets there is no agreed-upon dose. Empirically, doses suggested for people are used or modified for the veterinary patient.

Side Effects

Bee pollen and bee-related products are considered very safe. Allergic reactions are the most common side effect.

Contraindications

Bee products should not be used in patients with known allergies to bees, bee products, or poplar and conifer trees.[1]

Interactions

None reported.

References

1. Pizzorno J, Murray M. *Textbook of natural medicine*. 3rd ed. St. Louis (MO): Churchill Livingstone; 2006:767–8.

2. Wynn S, Marsden S. *Manual of natural veterinary medicine: science and tradition.* St. Louis (MO): Mosby; 2003:133, 189, 509.

3. Broadfoot PJ, Palmquist RE, Jonston K, et al. *Integrating complementary medicine into veterinary practice.* Goldstein R, ed. Blackwell; 2008:752. Available at: www.mediafire.com/?2s13ctmvv7tyb2k. Accessed January 15, 2012.

4. Fetrow CW, Avila J. *Professional's handbook of complementary & alternative medicines.* 3rd ed. Philadelphia (PA): Lippincott Williams & Wilkins; 2004:79–81, 675.

(*SACCHAROMYCES CEREVISIAE*)

Background

Brewer's yeast consists of the ground, dried cells of the fungus *Saccharomyces cerevisiae* and is used to ferment sugars into alcohol in the brewing of beer.[1] Brewer's yeast contains amino acids, vitamins, minerals, and high levels of chromium. The chromium is believed to help regulate blood sugar levels in humans with type 2 diabetes. Brewer's yeast is also thought to improve skin and hair health, control diarrhea, decrease serum cholesterol, and repel insects such as mosquitoes (because of its thiamin [vitamin B_1] content).[1] The insect-repelling properties make brewer's yeast popular in veterinary medicine as a natural alternative for flea control. The hypothesis is that insect-repelling components of brewer's yeast, such as thiamin, are excreted through sweat glands. Many owners report that brewer's yeast effectively controls fleas; however, these are only anecdotal reports. Controlled studies have demonstrated the ineffectiveness of brewer's yeast for controlling fleas in pets.[2,3] Nevertheless, administration of brewer's yeast is safe and its use as a natural method of flea control could be encouraged if the owner is concerned about the safety of medications marketed for flea control.

The quality of brewer's yeast varies depending upon the manufacturer. Some packaged brewer's yeasts are processed to remove the alcohol and chemical by-products that are left behind in the brewing process, which is thought to lower the nutritional quality of the yeast. High-quality brewer's yeast is grown on either molasses or sugar beets.

Indications

Suggested Uses in Humans
- Helps regulate blood sugar levels
- Improves the appearance of skin and hair
- Helps resolve diarrhea
- Controls hypercholesterolemia
- Functions as an insect repellent

Suggested Uses in Dogs and Cats
- Controls fleas

Recommended Doses

In both people and pets, the recommended dose varies from product to product. In the author's opinion, the recommended dose provided by the manufacturer is usually empirical, based on the thiamin (vitamin B_1) content of the supplement.

Side Effects

Brewer's yeast is considered very safe.

Contraindications

None reported.

Interactions

Although there do not appear to be any specific reports describing any interactions with brewer's yeast and other drugs, supplements, or herbs, there are some interactions for chromium and thiamine (both of which are found in brewer's yeast). For chromium, human male patients with hypertension exhibited improved high-density lipoprotein levels (HDL, "good" cholesterol) when taking chromium and beta-blockers (i.e., β-1-adrenoreceptor antagonists). In addition, chromium supplementation may decrease the development of steroid-induced (oral corticosteroid) diabetes. Further, chromium is believed to be involved in glucose and fat metabolism, and chromium supplementation may enhance the activity of insulin and oral hypoglycemic medications (but patients must be closely monitored for hypoglycemia). Finally, there is a small amount of indirect evidence that chromium picolinate (a specific form of chromium) can increase the synthesis of serotonin (5-HT) from tryptophan in the brain to benefit individuals with depression.

For thiamine, several interactions are recognized. First, antacids are known to interfere with the absorption of thiamine. Second, broad-spectrum antibiotics can destroy the "good" bacteria (commensals) in the gastrointestinal system that produce B vitamins, including thiamine; however, thiamine can interfere with the pharmacokinetics of the antibiotic tetracycline. Thiamine supplementation should therefore be avoided with tetracyclines. Third, thiamine can interfere with the chemotherapeutic agent 5-fluorouracil (5-FU) and should therefore be avoided during treatment. Fourth, furosemide and other loop diuretics can increase the excretion of thiamine. If the diuretics are administered for patients with heart failure, thiamine deficiency can contribute to cardiac insufficiency and worsen congestive heart failure. Coadministration of thiamine with diuretics is indicated. Fifth, administration of tricyclic antidepressants concurrently with thiamine results in improved responses. Sixth, anticonvulsants such as phenytoin can deplete thiamine. Supplementation is warranted.[4]

References

1. Fetrow CW, Avila J. *Professional's handbook of complementary & alternative medicines.* 3rd ed. Philadelphia (PA): Lippincott Williams & Wilkins; 2004:132–4.

2. Baker NF, Farver TB. Failure of brewer's yeast as a repellant to fleas on dogs. J *Am Vet Med Assoc* 1983;183(2):212–4.

3. Wynn S, Marsden S. *Manual of natural veterinary medicine: science and tradition.* St. Louis (MO): Mosby; 2003:142–3.

4. Stargrove M, Treasure J, McKee D. *Herb, nutrient, and drug interactions: clinical implications and therapeutic strategies.* St. Louis (MO): Mosby Elsevier; 2008:253–62.

CARNITINE

Background

Carnitine is an amino acid (a building block for proteins) found in high concentration in the heart and skeletal muscles, liver, and kidneys.[1] The body can synthesize carnitine from lysine and methionine and is therefore not an essential nutrient. Carnitine can also be obtained through the diet and is mainly found in foods of animal origin, such as meat, milk, eggs, and dairy products.[1] As a supplement, carnitine is available as L-carnitine, propionyl-L-carnitine, and L-acetylcarnitine (LAC), the latter of which has been used in patients with Alzheimer's disease.[1,2]

Carnitine acts a carrier for long-chain fatty acids and acyl-coenzyme A compounds (which are involved in energy production).[1] Specifically, carnitine transports these compounds into the mitochondria (special energy-producing organelles found inside cells), especially in skeletal and cardiac muscle, where they are oxidized to produce energy.[1] This explains how carnitine may increase endurance and improve cardiac performance.[1,3,4] In addition, carnitine supports hepatic detoxification and excretion of toxins/drugs/chemicals, helps dispose of glucose, improves insulin resistance, and plays an important role in the synthesis and release of the potent neurotransmitter acetylcholine, which is important for nerve transmission.[1] A number of clinical trials have also demonstrated that carnitine improves both angina and heart disease.[2]

Indications

Suggested Uses in Humans

- Improves/protects against heart disease (e.g., angina, myocardial insufficiency, arrhythmias, atherosclerosis, etc.)
- Enhances physical endurance
- Helps patients with Alzheimer's disease
- Facilitates weight loss

Suggested Uses in Dogs and Cats

- Improves/protects against heart disease
- Supports cognitive function
- Accelerates weight loss in cats[3]

Recommended Doses

In humans, 1,500–4,000 mg/day in three divided doses is recommended.[1] In dogs with heart disease, 50–100 mg/kg q 8 hr has been used.[3] In the author's experience, 100–2,000 mg/day in divided doses is appropriate for heart disease.

Side Effects

Even at high doses, L-carnitine is considered a very safe supplement with no significant side effects.[1] In humans, reported minor side effects include nausea and vomiting and sleeplessness if taken at night.[1] D-carnitine and products containing both forms (DL-carnitine) should be avoided as the D form is not active and may block the action of L-carnitine, producing signs of carnitine deficiency.[1]

Contraindications

Humans with low thyroid levels or hypothyroidism might consider avoiding carnitine supplementation, as it may impair the action of thyroid hormone.[1,3] Similar precautions might also apply to dogs with hypothyroidism.

Interactions

There are several important interactions worthy of mention. For example, L-carnitine may prevent or reduce cardiotoxicity associated with the administration of anthracycline chemotherapy (such as with doxorubicin), may reduce (hepato)toxicity that can occur with retinoids, and may prevent hearing loss when administered with aminoglycosides, especially gentamicin.[1] In patients with hyperthyroidism, carnitine may partially block the activity of thyroid hormone, and a positive additive (synergistic) effect occurs when L-carnitine supplementation is given to patients taking nitrates for cardiac disease.[1] Carnitine supplementation may be helpful in patients treated with anticonvulsants to prevent carnitine depletion.[1] Improved memory and metabolic function may occur in patients treated with L-carnitine and α-lipoic acid (ALA).[1] Patients with heart disease may benefit from a synergistic combination of supplements, including carnitine, coenzyme Q_{10} (CoQ10), fish oil, taurine, and hawthorn.[1] Finally, when given with choline, carnitine may help with hepatic lipidosis (250–500 mg carnitine q 24 hr).[3]

References

1. Stargrove M, Treasure J, McKee D. Herb, nutrient, and drug interactions: clinical implications and therapeutic strategies. St. Louis (MO): Mosby Elsevier; 2008:661–76.

2. Pizzorno J, Murray M. Textbook of natural medicine. 3rd ed. St. Louis (MO): Churchill Livingstone Elsevier; 2005:813–8.

3. Wynn S, Marsden S. Manual of natural veterinary medicine: science and tradition. St. Louis (MO): Mosby; 2003:81–91, 200, 248, 323.

4. Broadfoot PJ, Palmquist RE, Jonston K, et al. Integrating complementary medicine into veterinary practice. Goldstein R, ed. Blackwell; 2008:209, 216, 225. Available at: www.mediafire.com/?2s13ctmvv7tyb2k. Accessed January 15, 2012.

CHOLINE/PHOSPHATIDYLCHOLINE

Background

Choline is a nitrogen-containing essential nutrient that is critical for normal cell membrane structure and function. It is used to synthesize acetylcholine, an important neurotransmitter involved in nerve signaling.[1,2] In the diet, choline is predominantly found in phosphatidylcholine and lecithin, which are found in milk, eggs, liver, and peanuts.[1,3] Choline is a "methyl donator" (a methyl group is one carbon atom bound to three hydrogen atoms) and can therefore convert homocysteine to methionine, which may reduce the risk of cardiovascular disease (by lowering homocysteine levels).[2] Studies have shown that choline supplementation helps improve memory in Alzheimer's patients and the elderly and may also help patients with other brain-related disorders or conditions.[1] This is presumably attributable to the fact that, as mentioned above, choline is converted to acetylcholine in the brain.[1] Choline has also demonstrated some anticonvulsant properties.[1] In animals, choline supplementation may prevent fatty liver syndrome (in diabetics)[4] and may help prevent or treat cognitive disorder.[4] Choline is also believed to support liver function; reduce insulin requirements in diabetics; function as a constituent of plasmalogens (long fat chain containing phosphorus), which are abundant in mitochondria and sphingomyelin (a type of fat found in high concentrations in the lining of nerves); and reduce seizure frequency.[3]

Indications

Specific Uses in People
- Improves signs of Alzheimer's disease
- Supports patients with liver disease

Specific Uses in Dogs and Cats
- Helps with cognitive disorders
- Supports patients with epilepsy
- Improves diabetes
- Supports patients with liver disease

Recommended Doses

In people, the recommended dose of choline is 500–1,000 mg q 24 hr.[1] In dogs and cats, 20–40 mg/animal administered q 12–24 hr is recommended for cognitive disorders.[3] Choline can also be administered at a dose of 10–15 mg/0.45 kg body weight q 24 hr.[4] When choline is supplied as lecithin, the dose is either 1.23 mL (¼ teaspoon)/11.34 kg body weight q 12 hr or 1 g/9.1 kg body weight q 24 hr.[3,5]

Side Effects

Supplementation with choline is very safe. In dogs and cats, rare instances of excitability/nervousness have been reported, which can be resolved by lowering the dose.[3] In the author's experience, other side effects (which are only rarely reported in humans taking large doses >3.5 g/day) include hypotension, gastrointestinal discomfort, increased salivation, decreased appetite, sweating, and a "fishy" body odor because of the excessive production and excretion of trimethylamine, a metabolite of choline.

Contraindications

None reported.

Interactions

None reported.

References

1. Pizzorno J, Murray M. *Textbook of natural medicine*. 3rd ed. St. Louis (MO): Churchill Livingstone; 2005:817, 853, 856, 1603, 1654.

2. Hand M, Thatcher C, Remillard R, et al. *Small animal clinical nutrition*. 5th ed. Topeka (KS): Mark Morris Institute; 2010:93–4.

3. Messonnier SP. *The natural health bible for dogs & cats: your A–Z guide to over 200 herbs, vitamins, and supplements*. New York: Three Rivers Press; 2001:56–7, 233.

4. Wynn S, Marsden S. *Manual of natural veterinary medicine: science and tradition*. St. Louis (MO): Mosby; 2003:323.

5. Broadfoot PJ, Palmquist RE, Jonston K, et al. *Integrating complementary medicine into veterinary practice*. Goldstein R, ed. Blackwell; 2008:541. Available at: www .mediafire.com/?2s13ctmvv7tyb2k. Accessed January 15, 2012.

CHONDROITIN

(CHONDROITIN SULFATE, CHONDROITIN-4-SULFATE, CHONDROITIN-6-SULFATE)

Background

Chondroitin sulfate (CS) is a glycosaminoglycan (GAG), which is a long chain of disaccharides (sugar molecules) linked together and sulfated at either the fourth or sixth carbon atom (hence chondroitin-4-sulfate and chondroitin-6-sulfate).[1,2] CS is found in the articular cartilage that lines the ends of bones within joints. It is the most abundant GAG in the body, located in a variety of connective tissues. In cartilage, CS absorbs water and holds nutrients, enhancing the thickness and elasticity of cartilage and increasing the ability of the cartilage to absorb and distribute compressive forces during locomotion. CS also stimulates chondrocytes (cells in articular cartilage) to synthesize collagen and proteoglycans, enhances hyaluronic acid production, and inhibits degradative enzymes that break down cartilage and synovial fluid.[1] In articular cartilage, CS is synthesized and secreted by chondrocytes.

Animal cartilage is one of the only dietary sources of CS.[3] Nutritional supplements containing CS are therefore derived from animal cartilage, such as bovine trachea or shark and fish cartilage. Even though CS is a large molecule, studies show it is absorbed from the digestive system.[4] However, low-molecular-weight supplements are preferred when available because of their superior bioavailability.[3]

Indications

Suggested Uses in Humans
- Manages or prevents osteoarthritis

Suggested Uses in Dogs and Cats
- Manages or prevents osteoarthritis

Recommended Doses

In humans, the typical dose of CS is 300–600 mg q 8–24 hr.[2] The typical dose for dogs >22.7 kg is approximately 800 mg q 12–24 hr and approximately 200–400 mg q 12–24 hr for small and medium-sized dogs and cats.[5] In general, CS is not usually the sole supplement for pets with OA. Typically, joint supplements contain CS as well as other ingredients such as glucosamine and methylsulfonylmethane (MSM). Quality joint supplements should deliver these doses of CS regardless of the other ingredients included in the supplement.

Side Effects

Chondroitin is considered a safe supplement. Clinical reports of adverse reactions in dogs and cats are lacking. In humans, there are rare reports in people of gastrointestinal side effects such as diarrhea, constipation, abdominal pain, and very rarely headache, edema/swelling of the legs and eyelids, heart arrhythmias, and hair loss.[6]

Contraindications

In canine experiments, decreased red blood cell counts, white blood cell counts, and platelet counts occurred after 30 days of administration, but these side effects are not typically reported in clinical practice and the significance is unknown.[7] Nevertheless, naturopathic doctors for human patients often suggest avoiding chondroitin-containing supplements for short periods of time before and after surgery and in patients at risk for bleeding (e.g., hemophiliacs and individuals prescribed anticoagulants).[8]

There is some preliminary evidence suggesting that chondroitin sulfate supplements should be avoided in people (and probably pets) either at risk or diagnosed with certain cancers (e.g., prostate). This is because nonsulfated chondroitin sulfate is thought to play a role in the growth and spread of certain cancer cells.[9] Other joint supplements, such as those containing glucosamine sulfate or hyaluronic acid, can be used safely in patients with these conditions.[2]

Interactions

Chondroitin is often included in glucosamine-containing nutritional supplements. Although clinical studies are lacking, there are some *in vitro* data that suggest that using CS and glucosamine together achieves better results than using either alone.[1,2,8,10] In addition, primary research shows that coadministration of chondroitin sulfate supplements with platinum-based chemotherapy drugs (such as cisplatin) may decrease kidney toxicity from the chemotherapy drugs without decreasing their effectiveness.[1,2] There is also an important interaction between CS and NSAIDs. Patients with OA might require lower doses of NSAIDs, which is beneficial for the patient considering the cost and potential adverse reactions associated with NSAID administration.[1]

References

1. Stargrove M, Treasure J, McKee D. *Herb, nutrient, and drug interactions: clinical implications and therapeutic strategies.* St. Louis (MO): Mosby Elsevier; 2008:725–9.

2. Pizzorno J, Murray M. Textbook of natural medicine. 3rd ed. St. Louis (MO): Churchill Livingstone; 2006:615–6, 1966–7.

3. Pizzorno J, Murray M, Joiner-Bey H. The clinician's handbook of natural medicine. 2nd ed. St. Louis (MO): Churchill Livingstone; 2008:559.

4. Wynn S, Marsden S. *Manual of natural veterinary medicine: science and tradition.* St. Louis (MO): Mosby; 2003:369.

5. Messonnier SP. *The natural health bible for dogs & cats: your A–Z guide to over 200 herbs, vitamins, and supplements.* New York: Three Rivers Press; 2001:14, 181.

6. Sawitzke AD, Shi H, Finco MF, et al. Clinical efficacy and safety over two years use of glucosamine, chondroitin sulfate, their combination, celecoxib or placebo taken to treat osteoarthritis of the knee: a GAIT report. Ann Rheum Dis 2010;69:1459–64. Available at: http://www.ncbi.nlm.nih.gov/pmc/articles/PMC3086604/pdf/nihms267850.pdf. Accessed February 19, 2010.

7. McNamara PS, Barr SC, Erb HN. Hematologic, hemostatic, and biochemical effects in dogs receiving an oral chondroprotective agent for thirty days. *Am J Vet Res* 1996;57:1390–4.

8. Fetrow CW, Avila J. *Professional's handbook of complementary & alternative medicines.* 3rd ed. Philadelphia (PA): Lippincott Williams & Wilkins; 2004:205–9.

9. Teng YH, Tan PH, Chia SJ, et al. Increased expression of non-sulfated chondroitin correlates with adverse clinicopathological parameters in prostate cancer. *Mod Pathol* 2008;21(7):893–901.

10. Graeser AC, Giller K, Wiegand H, et al. Synergistic chondroprotective effect of alpha-tocopherol, ascorbic acid, and selenium as well as glucosamine and chondroitin on oxidant induced cell death and inhibition of matrix metalloproteinase-3—studies in cultured chondrocytes. *Molecules* 2009;15:27–39.

Background

Coenzyme Q$_{10}$ (CoQ10) is an antioxidant synthesized in most tissues in the body. The highest concentrations are in the heart, kidneys, liver, and pancreas.[1,2] In the diet, CoQ10 is found in foods such as organ meats, poultry, fish, meat, nuts, soybean oil, canola oil, fruits, vegetables, dairy products, and eggs.[2]

CoQ10 is one of several fat-soluble coenzymes used in electron transport in mitochondria—small organelles inside cells that produce energy. CoQ10 located in the inner mitochondrial membrane is required for the conversion of energy from carbohydrates and fats in the synthesis of adenosine triphosphate (ATP, energy).[2] Because CoQ10 is involved in reduction/oxidation reactions (i.e., able to accept and donate electrons), it can prevent the depletion of substrates required for the synthesis of ATP and protects cell membranes and DNA from oxidative damage and tissue from ischemic cellular damage.[1,2]

Deficiencies of CoQ10 levels can occur (in people) for the following reasons: failure of biosynthesis caused by a gene mutation; inhibition of biosynthesis by statins, which are used to reduce cholesterol levels in people; aging; diabetes; and cancer.[1,2]

Studies in people with hypertension showed a reduction in systolic blood pressure when administered CoQ10. Benefits of CoQ10 therapy are reported in people with heart failure (via increased left ventricular ejection fraction [a measure of how much blood is being pumped out of the heart], increased cardiac output and stroke volume, positive inotropy, and vasodilation).[1] CoQ10 also increases circulating immunoglobulin levels (IgG) and infection fighting CD4+ cells in the blood.[2] Considering the potential infection-fighting properties of CoQ10, there is also some evidence that it may help in gingivitis and stomatitis and may be useful for immunodeficiencies.[1,3] Because of its role in enhancing immune function, CoQ10 has been considered a possible anticancer agent in people (e.g., prostate cancer).[2] CoQ10 is a powerful antioxidant and holds therapeutic potential in the treatment of Parkinson's disease. Patients with diabetes mellitus have low CoQ10 levels, potentially because of mitochondrial dysfunction.[4]

CoQ10 supplements are available in two forms: fully oxidized ubiquinone and ubiquinol (the active reduced metabolite containing two hydroxyl groups). Most CoQ10 supplements use the more stable ubiquinone form, although a new patented human product utilizes stabilized ubiquinol. Studies in people and laboratory animals show that lower doses of the ubiquinol form can be used to achieve therapeutic blood levels. Ubiquinol is better absorbed and lasts in the body longer (is metabolized and excreted less quickly) than ubiquinone.

Indications

Suggested Uses in Humans

- Improves cardiovascular diseases (e.g., cardiomyopathy, angina, arrhythmias, following cardiac surgeries, mitral valve disease)
- Helps manage hypertension
- Acts as an anticancer agent
- Improves diabetes mellitus
- Helps gingivitis/periodontal disease
- Supports patients with immune disorders (e.g., HIV)
- Helps Parkinson's disease
- Assists geriatric patients

Suggested Uses in Pets

- Improves cardiovascular diseases (as described above for humans) and hypertension
- Acts as an anticancer agent
- Helps gingivitis/periodontal disease
- Supports geriatric patients
- Improves immune dysfunction
- Controls diabetes mellitus, hyperthyroidism, and hypothyroidism
- Improves muscular conditions such as degenerative myelopathy

Recommended Doses

In people, the recommended dose is 50–300 mg/day given in divided doses (e.g., 30–60 mg q 8–12 hr).[1] In pets, a reported dose for dogs and cats is 2–20 mg/kg/day in divided doses.[3] In the author's experience, however, a typical clinical dose is 2–4 mg/kg/day in divided doses. It is generally recommended that CoQ10 be taken with a meal or small amount of oil-containing fat because it is a fat-soluble supplement and will be better absorbed.[2]

Side Effects

CoQ10 is a very safe supplement. No significant adverse effects of toxicities have been reported in people or pets taking the recommended doses. In people, rare side effects include mild nausea, anorexia, vomiting, diarrhea, and flu-like symptoms.[2]

Contraindications

None reported.

Interactions

A number of important interactions are worth mentioning here. First, beta-blocking drugs inhibit mitochondrial CoQ10 activity to various degrees. Supplementation with CoQ10 may therefore be beneficial for patients prescribed beta-blockers.[2] Second, phenothiazines and related psychoactive medications may depress the myocardium (by inhibiting energy production). Supplementation with CoQ10 may be beneficial for these patients because it is involved in energy production.[2] Third, aglycone I, the major metabolite of anthracycline chemotherapeutic agents such as doxorubicin (but not liposome-encapsulated doxorubicin), exhibits negligible cardiotoxicity and generates free radicals through an iron-dependent process. Oxidative damage ensues, resulting in both acute and chronic cardiotoxicity. Anthracyclines also cause a reduction in the CoQ10 levels in mitochondrial (energy-producing organelles inside cells) membranes and inhibit the mitochondrial synthesis of CoQ10 and CoQ10-dependent enzymes. Supplementation with CoQ10 before, during, and after use of chemotherapeutic anthracyclines can prevent or reduce cardiotoxicity.[2] Fourth, statin drugs (HMG-CoA reductase inhibitors, chemicals that help reduce cholesterol) reduce CoQ10 levels because cholesterol and CoQ10 share the same biochemical pathway for their formation. Side effects caused by statin administration may occur as a result of decreased CoQ10 levels. Supplementation with CoQ10 may be warranted.[2] Fifth, in diabetic patients, some oral hypoglycemic agents may reduce already low CoQ10 levels, which might be abrogated by CoQ10 supplementation.[2] Sixth, tricyclic antidepressants may result in CoQ10 deficiency causing cardiotoxicity, which may be reversed with supplementation.[2] Seventh, CoQ10 and vitamin K share a similar chemical structure, making it theoretically possible that CoQ10 might interfere with warfarin or other vitamin K antagonist anticoagulants. Patients taking vitamin K antagonist anticoagulants should be monitored if they are also receiving CoQ10.[2] Eighth, patients taking levothyroxine (or other thyroid hormones) require monitoring if supplemented with CoQ10 as hormone levels might be impacted by supplementation. Ninth, and finally, a positive additive effect may occur with concomitant administration of L-carnitine and CoQ10.[2]

References

1. Fetrow CW, Avila J. *Professional's handbook of complementary & alternative medicines.* 3rd ed. Philadelphia (PA): Lippincott Williams & Wilkins; 2004:220–4.

2. Stargrove M, Treasure J, McKee D. *Herb, nutrient, and drug interactions: clinical implications and therapeutic strategies.* St. Louis (MO): Mosby Elsevier; 2008:732–45.

3. Wynn S, Marsden S. *Manual of natural veterinary medicine: science and tradition.* St. Louis (MO): Mosby; 2003:80, 189.

4. Pizzorno J, Murray M. *Textbook of natural medicine.* 3rd ed. St. Louis (MO): Churchill Livingstone; 2005:859–61.

Background

Historically, silver was used as a germicidal agent. Colloidal silver, a suspension of tiny silver particles suspended in a liquid, has been marketed as an effective alternative to conventional antimicrobials for a variety of conditions. Colloidal silver is available for oral use (for various internal infections) or topically for use on wounds (including ophthalmic and otic uses). There are numerous anecdotal reports regarding the efficacy of colloidal silver for various infectious conditions; however, these claims have not been substantiated or proven in controlled studies.[1,2]

The use of colloidal silver supplements for medicinal purposes is not supported by the U.S. Food and Drug Administration (FDA).[2] Specifically, no colloidal silver ingredients or products are considered either safe or effective, and the FDA has taken serious action against many companies for making unsubstantiated drug claims for their over-the-counter (OTC) colloidal silver products. According to the FDA's website, "None of the silver salts evaluated as part of the FDA's OTC drug review was found to be generally recognized as safe and effective for its intended use(s). FDA is not aware of any substantial scientific evidence that supports the use of OTC colloidal silver ingredients or silver salts for disease conditions."[3]

The FDA issued a final ruling in 1999 on colloidal silver products categorizing colloidal silver as an unclassified drug. Therefore, any colloidal silver products marketed as having medicinal properties are in violation of federal law.[3] However, because silver is a natural substance, not a controlled substance, substances labeled as a dietary supplement without drug-like claims are available.

In the author's experience, there are pet owners who insist on using colloidal silver products. Topical products applied to wounds may be effective for controlling infections and assisting in healing and are likely safe. Ingestion of oral products and the use of ophthalmic products (to the eyes) is of more concern as these colloidal silver products can cause irritation or toxicity.[4] Erring on the side of safety prevents most doctors (human and veterinary) from prescribing oral and ophthalmic products containing colloidal silver.

Silver binds to proteins to denature them by forming hemisilver complexes with certain functional groups on the proteins (such as sulfhydryl, amino, carboxyl, phosphate, and imidazole groups). Silver also alters the activities of certain enzymes such as lactate dehydrogenase and glutathione peroxidase, which causes lipid peroxidation (e.g., in cell membranes).[4]

Indications
Suggested Uses in Humans
- Helps various topical infections, including otitis
- Ophthalmic conditions

Suggested Uses in Dogs and Cats
- Helps various topical infections, including otitis
- Ophthalmic conditions

Recommended Doses
There is no recommended dose for colloidal silver and there is no standardization of products among manufacturers.[1] In dogs and cats, topical application of small amounts of colloidal silver as part of the treatment of minor wounds appears to be safe. In the author's experience, many pet owners have reported no serious side effects when using colloidal silver orally per package instructions.

Side Effects
Side effects have been reported in people using colloidal silver products that either contained high doses of silver or were used for extended periods of time.[5-8] Potential side effects following oral administration include status epilepticus (seizures), renal damage, headache, and fatigue, among others. Skin irritation has been reported following topical use as well as argyria—a permanent blue-gray discoloration of the skin, nails, and organs because of the buildup of silver in the body.[2,5,6] Because of the lack of established effectiveness and potential toxicity of these products, colloidal silver products are generally not recommended without strict medical supervision. Owners are encouraged to wear gloves when applying topical products and when administering oral supplements containing colloidal silver. It may also be prudent to prevent pets from licking topical colloidal silver products (e.g., by using an Elizabethan collar).

Contraindications

None reported. Because of safety concerns, colloidal silver products should not be used in either infants or pregnant or lactating women. Similar precautions likely apply to pets.

Interactions

Colloidal silver products may interact with some medications, including penicillamine, quinolones, tetracycline, and thyroxine.[2]

References

1. Mayo Clinic. Consumer health. Question: colloidal silver: is it safe or effective? Available at: www.mayoclinic.com/health/colloidal-silver/AN01682. Accessed January 9, 2012.

2. National Institutes of Health. National Center for Complementary and Alternative Medicine (NCCAM). Backgrounder: colloidal silver products. Available at: http://nccam.nih.gov/health/silver/. Accessed January 9, 2012.

3. U.S. Food and Drug Administration. Colloidal silver not approved. Available at: http://www.fda.gov/AnimalVeterinary/NewsEvents/CVMUpdates/ucm127976.htm. Accessed February 19, 2012.

4. Memorial Sloan-Kettering Cancer Center. Colloidal silver. herbs, botanicals & other products. Available at: http://www.mskcc.org/cancer-care/herb/colloidal-silver. Accessed March 12, 2012.

5. Agency for Toxic Substances and Disease Registry (ATSDR). ToxFAQs for silver. Available at: http://www.atsdr.cdc.gov/toxfaqs/tf.asp?id=538&tid=97. Accessed January 9, 2012.

6. Fung MC, Bowen DL. Silver products for medical indications: risk-benefit assessment. *J Toxicol Clin Toxicol* 1996;34(1):119–26.

7. Gulbranson SH, Hud JA, Hansen RC. Argyria following the use of dietary supplements containing colloidal silver protein. *Cutis* 2000;66(5):373–4.

8. White JM, Powell AM, Brady K, et al. Severe generalized argyria secondary to ingestion of colloidal silver protein. *Clin Exp Dermatol* 2003;28(3):254–6.

Background

Colostrum, the first fluid secreted by the mammary glands immediately following parturition, contains infection-fighting antibodies, growth factors, nutrients, cytokines (inflammatory mediators), glycoproteins, lactoferrin, lactalbumin, leukocytes (infection-fighting white blood cells), lysozymes, vitamins, and insulin-like growth factors. These ingredients stimulate cell growth, tissue repair, and provide immune support to the recipient.[1,2] Colostrum also contains "transfer factors," which are small peptides (short proteins composed of amino acids) produced by a specific type of infection-fighting white blood cell.[3]

The level of immunoglobulins (antibodies) is approximately 100 times higher in bovine colostrum than in regular bovine milk, and bovine colostrum contains higher levels of immunoglobulins and growth factors than human milk. Cows are commonly used when making colostrum supplements. Most supplements are available as dried colostrum.[2] The immune and growth factors in colostrum, however, are easily destroyed by heat, making proper manufacturing essential if colostrum supplementation is to be of any benefit. When possible, independent assays should be available to ensure that the immune growth factors are still viable in the colostrum products selected. Standardization of colostrum products would be helpful to ensure quality.[2]

Colostrum supplementation is thought to improve intestinal health, balance intestinal flora, and improve digestion. It also can improve the immune status of the intestinal tract, which can be weakened by intestinal parasites.[3] Colostrum is also used for infections, cancers, as an antiaging product, and for diarrhea.[3] Colostrum may be beneficial in these conditions; more research is needed to confirm efficacy before widespread recommendations can be made (as with many nutritional supplements).

Indications

Suggested Uses in Humans

- Supports immune function
- Enhances recovery after exercise
- Decreases intestinal permeability (leakiness) that may occur after damage to intestinal cells by toxins, microorganisms, and medications

Suggested Uses in Pets
- Supports the immune system
- Enhances recovery after exercise
- Decreases intestinal permeability (leakiness) that may occur following damage to intestinal cells by toxins, microorganisms, and medications
- Controls intestinal parasites
- Helps patients with pancreatitis, periodontitis, and stomatitis

Recommended Doses
The dose typically varies with the product, as no standard dosing is available. In dogs and cats, 1.65 mL (⅓ teaspoon) of powdered colostrum/11.3 kg body weight *q* 12 hr is a recommended starting dose.[4]

Side Effects
Colostrum is considered a safe supplement.

Contraindications
None reported.

Interactions
None reported.

References
1. Hand M., Thatcher C, Remillard R., et al. *Small animal clinical nutrition.* 5th ed. Topeka (KS): Mark Morris Institute; 2010:244–6, 331–2.

2. Fetrow CW, Avila J. *Professional's handbook of complementary & alternative medicines.* 3rd ed. Philadelphia (PA): Lippincott Williams & Wilkins; 2004:230–3.

3. Memorial Sloan-Kettering Cancer Center. Transfer factor. About herbs, botanicals & other products. Available at: http://www.mskcc.org/cancer-care /herb/transfer-factor. Accessed March 12, 2012.

4. Broadfoot PJ, Palmquist RE, Jonston K, et al. *Integrating complementary medicine into veterinary practice.* Goldstein R, ed. Blackwell; 2008:294–8, 373–7, 626–8. Available at: www.mediafire.com/?2s13ctmvv7tyb2k. Accessed January 15, 2012.

DEHYDROEPIANDROSTERONE

(DHEA)

Background

DHEA (and its sulfated metabolite, DHEA-S) are among the most abundant naturally occurring steroids in the body.[1] DHEA is synthesized in the adrenal gland (located near the kidney), the central nervous system, gonads (testes and ovaries), skin, and gastrointestinal tract.[1-3] The exact role of DHEA remains largely unknown at this time, but DHEA does serve as a precursor for the synthesis of >50 different hormones, including androgenic and estrogenic steroids.[1,2] Peak production of DHEA by the adrenal gland occurs between 25 years and 30 years of age in humans. Levels decline with age and possibly during times of either stress or severe illness.[3]

DHEA administration has been suggested to prevent or reverse conditions associated with low endogenous DHEA levels, including aging, diabetes, cancer, and autoimmune diseases.[4] DHEA may also help with both hyper- and hypoadrenocorticism (Cushing's and Addison's disease, respectively), potentially improve mood and feelings of well-being in people with depression; and may reduce the risk of developing diabetes or enhance the treatment of patients with diabetes.[1,3,5]

Supplements are usually prepared from DHEA precursors isolated from wild yams or soy, which are then chemically synthesized into DHEA.[3]

Indications

Suggested Uses in Humans

- Slows the aging process
- Helps immune/autoimmune diseases and HIV/AIDS
- Supports patients with diabetes mellitus, Addison's disease (adrenal insufficiency, hypoadrenocorticism), hypogonadism, and menopause
- Helps patients with Alzheimer's disease

Suggested Uses in Dogs and Cats

- Supports cancer patients
- Helps patients with hyper- or hypoadrenocorticism

Recommended Doses

In healthy people, doses range from 10 to 30 mg/day, and people with autoimmune diseases may require as much as 50 mg *q* 12 hr. There is currently no agreed-upon dose, and most doctors recommend starting at a low dose, then adjusting the dose based on the patient's clinical response.[6]

In dogs and cats, a dose of 5 mg/9 kg of body weight *q* 24 hr is suggested, with a stated range of 5–50 mg *q* 24 hr. As with people, dividing the dose and administering *q* 12 hr may be preferred to maintain blood levels and more accurately reflect endogenous hormone secretion.[5]

Side Effects

DHEA is not considered appropriate for use in people under the age of 18 unless clinically applicable (e.g., adrenal insufficiency) because it may interfere with hormones involved in development.[2,6] The long-term safety has not been established through well-designed clinical studies in any species. DHEA is a precursor to a large number of hormones in the body and unintended side effects are certainly possible.[2,6] Side effects that have been reported in people include abnormal liver function, slightly decreased hemoglobin and red blood cell counts, hirsutism (excessive hair growth in women, masculinization of women), gynecomastia (abnormal development of large mammary glands in males), aggressiveness, fatigue, headache, irritability, insomnia, and nasal congestion.[3]

Contraindications

DHEA should not be used in patients with cancers under the influence of testosterone or estrogen, although the 7-keto variant of DHEA may be safe to use in these patients.[3] DHEA may be particularly beneficial in older patients; the elderly are more likely to have conditions such as benign prostatic hyperplasia and should be screened for these conditions before beginning DHEA supplementation.[3] Until more research is done, DHEA supplementation is not recommended for patients with insulin-dependent diabetes. If used, close supervision and regular monitoring are advocated.[3]

Interactions

DHEA should be avoided with benzodiazepines (e.g., diazepam [Valium®]) medications. This is because there is a potential for DHEA to inhibit the metabolism of benzodiazepines and for benzodiazepines to increase endogenous DHEA levels.[3] Close monitoring of patients taking anticoagulants is necessary as DHEA may affect coagulation.[3] Although anticonvulsant medications may lower serum DHEA levels, elevated DHEA levels that result from supplementation with DHEA may inhibit the therapeutic action of anticonvulsant medications. Caution should be used in patients coadministered DHEA and an anticonvulsant medication.[3]

Some positive interactions have also been described. There is a potential therapeutic benefit from DHEA supplementation with clonidine and fluoxetine.[2] Oral corticosteroid therapy lowers serum levels of both DHEA and DHEA-S. DHEA supplementation for patients on long-term corticosteroid therapy may therefore counteract some of the negative side effects of corticosteroid therapy (such as muscle wasting) without losing the benefits of corticosteroid therapy.[4] Combining DHEA with estrogen may enhance therapeutic efficacy and reduce side effects seen in women taking estrogen/progesterone as part of hormone replacement therapy. However, administering DHEA with estrogen has the potential to increase adverse effects resulting from elevated levels of either estrogen or DHEA. The same potential for reducing side effects and increasing efficacy as well as possibly producing adverse effects is also applicable to patients taking methyltestosterone and related medications.[2] Finally, DHEA may potentiate thyroid medications, potentially increasing the risk of thyrotoxicosis.[2] It is likely not recommended for use in cats with uncontrolled hyperthyroidism.

References

1. Pizzorno J, Murray M, Joiner-Bey H. *The clinician's handbook of natural medicine.* 2nd ed. St. Louis (MO): Churchill Livingstone; 2008:45.

2. Stargrove M, Treasure J, McKee D. *Herb, nutrient, and drug interactions: clinical implications and therapeutic strategies.* St. Louis (MO): Mosby Elsevier; 2008:746–56.

3. Fetrow CW, Avila J. *Professional's handbook of complementary & alternative medicines.* 3rd ed. Philadelphia (PA): Lippincott Williams & Wilkins; 2004:280–5.

4. Wynn S, Marsden S. *Manual of natural veterinary medicine: science and tradition.* St. Louis (MO): Mosby; 2003:200, 265, 272.

5. Broadfoot PJ, Palmquist RE, Jonston K, et al. *Integrating complementary medicine into veterinary practice*. Goldstein R, ed. Blackwell; 2008:21–2, 513, 515. Available at: www.mediafire.com/?2s13ctmvv7tyb2k. Accessed January 15, 2012.

6. Pizzorno J, Murray M. *Textbook of natural medicine*. 3rd ed. St. Louis (MO): Churchill Livingstone; 2006:899–904.

Background

DMG is synthesized in the body from the amino acid glycine. It is also synthesized from choline and betaine. Specifically, betaine has three methyl groups (one carbon atom with three hydrogen atoms). Once one of the methyl groups is removed, the remaining product is DMG. DMG is then oxidized to produce the amino acid glycine and two formaldehyde atoms. The formaldehyde atoms are used to produce folic acid (vitamin B_9).[1,2] The methyl groups of DMG are also used to produce other compounds, such as choline, S-adenosylmethionine (SAMe), methionine, hormones, neurotransmitters, and DNA.[3]

As an antioxidant, DMG offers protection from radiation therapy,[4] and may reverse some of the negative effects of autoimmune diseases.[3] DMG also exerts an anti-inflammatory effect and may be helpful in treating patients with inflammatory diseases such as osteoarthritis.[4] DMG may help patients improve their (athletic) performance and endurance,[2] improve circulatory and heart function, provide higher energy levels, and allow patients to eliminate or significantly reduce their cardiac medications.[3] DMG is considered an "anti-stress" compound that may be beneficial for any patient experiencing stress.[3] Studies have shown that DMG can improve the immune response by potentiating both cell-mediated and humoral immunity (the two main "branches" of the immune system), as well as stimulating the production of inflammatory mediators (cytokines) such as interferon, tumor necrosis factor, and various interleukins.[3] DMG is found in low levels in foods such as meats, seeds, and grains.[3]

Indications

Suggested Uses in Humans
- Supports the immune system
- Helps patients with cancer
- Fights infections

Suggested Uses in Pets
- Supports the immune system

- Helps patients with cancer
- Fights infections

Recommended Doses
Anecdotal doses of 100–200 mg *q* 6–8 hr have been recommended in humans. In dogs and cats, 450 mg/11.3 kg body weight *q* 12–24 hr is suggested.[4] In the author's experience, 125 mg/2.3–18.1 kg body weight *q* 12–24 hr may also be appropriate.

Side Effects
DMG is extremely safe.

Contraindications
None reported.

Interactions
None reported.

References
1. Pizzorno J, Murray M. *Textbook of natural medicine*. 3rd ed. St. Louis (MO): Churchill Livingstone; 2005:613, 1655.

2. Schoen AM, Wynn SG. *Complementary and alternative veterinary medicine: principles and practice*. St. Louis (MO): Mosby; 1998:36–7.

3. Kendall R. *Building wellness with DMG*. Topanga (CA): Freedom Press; 2003.

4. Broadfoot PJ, Palmquist RE, Jonston K, et al. *Integrating complementary medicine into veterinary practice*. Goldstein R, ed. Blackwell; 2008:509,722–3. Available at: www.mediafire.com/?2s13ctmvv7tyb2k. Accessed January 15, 2012.

(*ECHINACEA ANGUSTIFOLIA, E. PURPUREA, E. PALLIDA*)

Background

Echinacea nutritional supplements, usually made from the roots and flowers, are commonly used for immunomodulation (stimulation of the immune system).[1] Echinacea enhances cell-mediated immunity (especially phagocytosis, the "eating" of foreign organisms, such as bacteria or viruses, by infection-fighting white blood cells in the circulation).[1] Echinacea increases natural killer cell (a specific type of white blood cell that kills tumor cells and virus-containing cells) numbers and activity.[2] Echinacea also has antimicrobial activity and purportedly possesses anti-inflammatory properties and aids in wound healing.[1,3]

Echinacea contains a number of active ingredients, such as flavonoids (plant secondary metabolites), polysaccharides (long sugar chains), alkaloids (secondary metabolites), and caffeic acid (a product produced by plants with anticancer and anti-inflammatory properties) and its derivatives.[4]

In addition, echinacea may assist bone marrow recovery following myelosuppressive chemotherapies.[4]

Indications

Suggested Uses in Humans

- Fights infections (viral and bacterial infections, particularly upper respiratory tract infections, candidiasis)
- Supports patients with chemotherapy-induced immunosuppression
- Helps control (chronic) inflammatory conditions

Suggested Uses in Dogs and Cats

- Fights infections (viral and bacterial infections, particularly upper respiratory tract infections, candidiasis)

Recommended Doses

In humans, 1–5 g *q* 24 hr of the dried root, 2.5–6 g *q* 24 hr of the dried flowers, and 3–6 mL *q* 24 hr of a 1:1 fluid extract are recommended.

It should be noted that the dose may vary widely depending on the type and source of the echinacea.[4] In dogs and cats, 25–300 mg/kg in divided doses is recommended. Alternatively, 0.5–1.5 mL of a 1:2–1:3 tincture/10 kg divided daily is recommended.[1]

Side Effects

Echinacea is considered a safe herb when properly administered. Side effects are uncommon and can include minor gastrointestinal symptoms (which may be relieved by the coadministration of probiotics, in the author's opinion), increased urination, and mild allergic reactions. Rarely, severe allergic reactions occur in atopic human patients exposed to echinacea. This is thought to be an immunoglobulin E-mediated (type 1 allergic reaction, like peanut allergies) adverse drug reaction in susceptible individuals (such as those with allergies to other members of the daisy family).[5,6]

Contraindications

Echinacea should be avoided in patients allergic to the herb.[5] Echinacea use in patients with autoimmune diseases is controversial and should be used with caution in these patients.

Interactions

A number of important interactions have been reported. For example, echinacea may increase the anticancer effects of low-dose cyclophosphamide.[4] Echinacea can inhibit cytochrome enzyme 2C9 (CYP2C9), which means that patients supplemented with echinacea concomitantly with drugs that are metabolized by this enzyme (e.g., phenytonin, S-warfarin, sulfonylureas) may pose a potential risk. Further research is needed to determine the exact effects of echinacea on various drug-metabolizing enzymes.[4] Echinacea can also inhibit CYP1A2 and its use should be avoided in patients taking drugs metabolized by this enzyme (e.g., tacrine, theophylline, caffeine, tricyclic antidepressants).[4]

It is not recommended to use echinacea for >8 weeks at a time because of the possibility of hepatotoxicity because of the potential presence of trace amounts of hepatotoxic alkaloids.[5,6] However, the usual alkaloids found in the roots of echinacea lack the necessary ring structure to be hepatotoxic. Thus, using echinacea for extended periods of time is unlikely to cause hepatotoxicity.[6]

It has also been recommended not to administer echinacea for >8 weeks at a time because of the possibility of suppression of immune function (which is based on the German Commission E recommendation for short-term use because of immune stimulation in patients with autoimmune diseases such as systemic lupus erythematosus and rheumatoid arthritis). That said, there is no evidence of immunosuppression with long-term echinacea use in other individuals, and echinacea may be used for >8 weeks if needed.[1]

References

1. Wynn SG, Fougère B. *Veterinary herbal medicine*. St. Louis (MO): Elsevier; 2007:93–4, 295–6, 383–4, 538–40.

2. Broadfoot PJ, Palmquist RE, Jonston K, et al. *Integrating complementary medicine into veterinary practice*. Goldstein R, ed. Blackwell; 2008:660, 700, 708. Available at: www.mediafire.com/?2s13ctmvv7tyb2k. Accessed January 15, 2012.

3. Mills S, Bone K. *Principles and practice of phytotherapy: modern herbal medicine*. St. Louis (MO): Churchill Livingstone; 2000:354–61.

4. Stargrove M, Treasure J, McKee D. *Herb, nutrient, and drug interactions: clinical implications and therapeutic strategies*. St. Louis (MO): Mosby Elsevier; 2008:32–8.

5. Fetrow CW, Avila J. *Professional's handbook of complementary and alternative medicines*. 3rd ed. Philadelphia (PA): Lippincott Williams & Wilkins; 2004:293–9.

6. Pizzorno J, Murray M. *Textbook of natural medicine*. 3rd ed. St. Louis (MO): Churchill Livingstone; 2005:907–16.

(OMEGA-3 FATTY ACIDS, EICOSAPENTAENOIC ACID, DOCOSAHEXAENOIC ACID)

Background

Fish oil is one of the most commonly recommended supplements for both people and pets and is a popular source of omega-3 fatty acids. Other sources of omega-3 fatty acids are flax oil, wheat germ oil, and canola oil.[1] Fish oil contains docosahexaenoicacid (DHA) and eicosapentaenoic acid (EPA).[1,2] Omega-3 and omega-6 fatty acids (the numbers simply refer to where the carbon-carbon double bonds are in the molecules) are metabolized by the arachadonic acid pathway. Omega-6 fatty acids, which are found in warm-weather vegetable oils, produce pro-inflammatory mediators such as prostacyclin, prostaglandin E2, and thromboxane A2.[1] The principal metabolites derived from the metabolism of EPA and DHA, in contrast, tend to be anti-inflammatory.[1] The typical American diet contains more omega-6 fatty acids than omega-3 fatty acids. Because omega-6 and omega-3 fatty acids compete with each other to be converted to active metabolites (pro-inflammatory and anti-inflammatory) in the body, decreasing the intake of omega-6 fatty acids and/or increasing dietary omega-3 fatty acid levels (especially through supplementation with fish oil) is thought to be beneficial.[3] That said, the optimal ratio of omega-6:omega-3 fatty acids has not been conclusively determined (but most recommendations are for a ratio of ≤2.5:1).[4]

In addition to the effect of the generation of inflammatory mediators, a number of other beneficial effects of fish oil supplementation have been noted. EPA and DHA replace other fatty acids in cell membranes. As a result, fish oil improves blood-flow characteristics and decreases platelet aggregation that benefits patients with atherosclerosis and those at risk for strokes. DHA is concentrated in gray matter (in the brain) and the retina (in the eye) and plays a role in development (neurologic, cognitive, and behavioral).[1,3]

Fish oil has been shown to have a beneficial effect in people with bipolar disorder and depression,[5] may exhibit antithrombotic effects,[6] and is beneficial in the treatment of heart disease. Fish oil may reduce atherosclerosis, thrombosis, coronary heart disease, myocardial infarction, sudden cardiac death, and stroke.[3] Fish oil may reduce side effects of cancer chemotherapy (including cardiotoxicity) and radiation therapy, reduce the growth and metastasis of cancer, and reduce cachexia in undernourished patients.[1] In addition, fish oil may potentiate the cytotoxicity of certain chemotherapeutic agents (making them more effective).[1]

Fish oil may be beneficial in gastrointestinal diseases, including inflammatory bowel disease by modulating inflammation,[7] may cause a modest lowering of blood pressure,[5] and may be useful in people with hypertensive disorders.[3] In humans, fish oil is reportedly superior to statin therapy for lowering mortality in patients with cardiovascular disease despite having only modest effects on lipids. Fish oil may lower lipid levels (especially triglycerides) but may cause minor elevations in LDL concentration (the "bad" cholesterol).[1] Fish oil may be protective against gastrointestinal side effects induced by nonsteroidal anti-inflammatory drugs (such as aspirin).[1] Finally, fish oil can help with atopy, seborrhea, and psoriasis, presumably because (at least in part) of its anti-inflammatory properties.[5]

For supplements, fish oil tends to be derived from cold-water fish that are rich in EPA and DHA (e.g., wild salmon, mackerel, sardine, anchovy, and herring). Occasionally, cod liver is used as a source of fish oil. Wild fish tend to have higher concentrations of EPA and DHA than farm-raised fish because of their food source (processed fish food fed to farm-raised fish may not contain high levels of EPA and DHA and may have a different balance of fatty acids).[3]

To minimize oxidation, fish oil products should be kept refrigerated after opening.[1] Because the EPA in fish oil takes time to become incorporated into cell membranes, it may take 4–6 months or longer before a clinical improvement is noted.[3] Fish oil supplementation may produce better clinical improvement than flax oil or other ALA fatty acid supplements, as these other sources of fatty acids need to be metabolized to form EPA and DHA.

Indications

Suggested Uses in Humans

- Minimizes inflammation
- Helps patients with certain heart disease
- Supports patients with arthritis
- Helps control depression

Suggested Uses in Pets
- Minimizes inflammation
- Helps patients with certain heart disease
- Supports patients with arthritis
- Controls kidney disease
- Improves atopy/skin disorders

Recommended Doses

Dosing is based upon the EPA and DHA content and not the "fish oil" content. In general, 1,000 mg of fish oil contains 180 mg EPA and 120 mg DHA. Commercial products vary widely in their concentrations of EPA and DHA; it is important to read the label to determine how much EPA and DHA is in the supplement.[1]

In humans, clinical trials usually use 3,000–4,000 g of EPA plus DHA (or more) daily.[1] For general supplementation, usually 1,000–2,000 mg of EPA plus DHA is recommended/day.[1] For dogs and cats, between 250 mg and 1,000 mg/animal/day has been suggested.[2,6] In the author's experience, veterinarians typically recommend 250–500 mg q 8–12 hr in small dogs and cats, 500–1,000 mg q 8–12 hr in medium-breed dogs, and 1,000–2,000 mg q 8–12 hr in large- and giant-breed dogs.

Side Effects

Fish oil is generally considered to be very safe. The most commonly reported side effects are a generalized fishy body odor, belching, nausea, and loose stools. Gastrointestinal side effects can be minimized if fish oil supplements are taken with food. If side effects persist, lowering the dose of fish oil supplements usually resolves any side effects.[1] Skin rashes are rarely reported in people taking fish oil, as are reports of mild elevation in the liver enzyme alanine aminotransferase (ALT) in people.[1] Elevated blood glucose levels have been reported in humans taking >3,000 mg fish oil/day for extended periods of time.[1] Fish liver oils (cod liver oil), but not fish oils, contain high levels of vitamins A and D and toxicity could be an issue (e.g., nausea, vomiting, weakness, etc.).[1] Concerns exist regarding heavy metal accumulation, especially methylmercury, in fish; however, fish meat contains considerably more toxins than fish oil. In fact, fish oil is generally considered to be free from heavy metal contamination, and molecular distillation is used to remove polychlorinated biphenyls (PCBs) and other toxins from fish oil. Nonrefined fish oil may contain pesticides or pollutants, and toxins have been found in both farm-raised and wild fish.[1]

Fish oil may decrease platelet aggregation,[6] prolong bleeding time, increase fibrinolysis, and diminish von Willebrand factor,[1] all of which theoretically could increase the risk of bleeding in supplemented patients. In particular, there have been some reports of serious, even fatal, intracranial bleeds in people taking high doses of fish oil (usually ≥9 g fish oil/day), especially when these high doses of fish oil are combined with other drugs (nonsteroidal anti-inflammatory drugs, warfarin) or supplements (garlic, *Ginkgo biloba*, ginseng) that also exert anticoagulant activities.[1]

Contraindications

Although fish oil is considered safe, patients with cardiac arrhythmias need to be monitored closely when introducing supplemental fish oil. Some patients have an increased chance of developing atrial fibrillation.[1] Similarly, patients with diabetes, hypertension, and other cardiovascular diseases should be closely monitored. Patients with hyperlipidemia may be at risk of spontaneous bleeding and the cumulative dose of the fat-soluble vitamins (especially A and D).[1]

Interactions

Fish oil can potentiate the cytotoxicity of vincristine, cisplatin, and doxorubicin.[1] Administering fish oil with cyclosporine after organ transplant can improve renal function and decrease hypertension.[1] Fish oil administered with statin medications achieves greater reductions in cholesterol and triglyceride concentrations than when either agent is used alone.[1] Extremely high doses of fish oil may increase bleeding, especially in patients taking anticoagulant medications and supplements (>9 g fish oil/day).[1] Vitamin E is typically added to official products to protect against oxidative damage and because long-term use of high doses of fish oil may deplete vitamin E from the body.[3] There is also limited evidence suggesting that fish oil may help reduce the rate of renal injury in patients with Immunoglobulin A (IgA) nephropathy, and may be beneficial when administered with angiotensin-converting enzyme (ACE) inhibitors.[1] Finally, fish oil can be coadministered with anticonvulsant medications to potentially reduce seizure frequency.[1]

References

1. Stargrove M, Treasure J, McKee D. *Herb, nutrient, and drug interactions: clinical implications and therapeutic strategies.* St. Louis (MO): Mosby Elsevier; 2008:783–806.

2. Broadfoot PJ, Palmquist RE, Jonston K, et al. *Integrating complementary medicine into veterinary practice.* Goldstein R, ed. Blackwell; 2008:210, 545, 548. Available at: www.mediafire.com/?2s13ctmvv7tyb2k. Accessed January 15, 2012.

3. Pizzorno J, Murray M. *Textbook of natural medicine.* 3rd ed. St. Louis (MO): Churchill Livingstone; 2005:946–61, 2098–2100.

4. Wander RC, Hall JA, Gradin JL, et al. The ratio of dietary (n-6) to (n-3) fatty acids influences immune system function, eicosanoid metabolism, lipid peroxidation and vitamin E status in aged dogs. J Nutr 1997;127(6):1198–205.

5. Pizzorno J, Murray M, Joiner-Bey H. *The clinician's handbook of natural medicine.* 2nd ed. St. Louis (MO): Churchill Livingstone; 2008:22, 23, 93, 350, 488, 716, 702–7.

6. Wynn S, Marsden S. *Manual of natural veterinary medicine: science and tradition.* St. Louis (MO): Mosby; 2003:286–7, 378, 523, 532.

7. Hand M, Thatcher C, Remillard R, et al. *Small animal clinical nutrition.* 5th ed. Topeka (KS): Mark Morris Institute; 2010:909–16.

(LINSEED OIL, *LINUM USITATISSIMUM*)

Background

Flaxseed and flaxseed oil contain large amounts of unsaturated fatty acids, including linoleic acid (LA), alpha-linolenic acid (ALA), and oleic acid.[1] Most activities of flaxseed oil are similar to those of fish oil, and the same uses apply (see the "Fish Oil" section for more detailed information). In addition, flaxseed is thought to help with constipation,[2] and studies in mice have shown that lignans in flaxseed can be helpful for cancer, especially breast and lung cancer.[3–5] Flaxseed may also have weak antiestrogenic, estrogenic,[3,4,6] and steroid-like activity.[1]

Flaxseed oil should be refrigerated to prevent breakdown of the essential fatty acids. Ground flaxseeds should be consumed within 24 hours, as their unsaturated fatty acids degrade through oxidation.[7]

Indications

Suggested Uses in Humans

- Helps resolve constipation
- Improves dry skin
- Benefits patients with diabetes
- Controls cardiovascular disease, hypertension
- Manages inflammatory bowel disease and irritable bowel syndrome
- Decreases serum cholesterol and low-density lipoproteins ("bad" cholesterol) levels
- Improves signs of menopause
- Supports cancer patients

Suggested Uses in Dogs and Cats

- Improves skin and hair coat
- Supports cancer patients

Recommended Doses

In humans flaxseed is generally administered as an oil (liquid form) to deliver 7–14 g ALA/day. Typically this is achieved by administering 15–30 mL (1–2 tablespoons) of flaxseed oil *q* 8–12 hr.

Capsules rather than liquid can be used but typically contain only 500 mg of ALA/1,000 mg capsule, requiring numerous capsules to be taken daily to achieve this dose.[7] In dogs and cats, 5 mL (1 teaspoon) of flax oil/11.3 kg body weight q 12–24 hr is recommended.[5] In the author's experience, 5–15 mL (1 teaspoon – 1 tablespoon)/11.3 kg body weight of freshly ground flaxseed q 12–24 hr is also recommended.

Side Effects

Flaxseed is very safe. Rare side effects include diarrhea, flatulence, and nausea. Allergic reactions can occur in patients who are allergic to flax.[1] Immature and raw seedpods are poisonous because of increased levels of cyanogenic nitrates,[1] which can result in signs of chronic cyanide poisoning (e.g., weakness, hypothyroidism).

Contraindications

Because of the phytoestrogen content there is a concern about flax administration in pregnant or lactating patients;[1] however, this has not been fully demonstrated. Animal studies have suggested possible side effects. Nonetheless, many pregnant and lactating women do consume flax products without noticeable effect in themselves or their infants.[7] Administration of flaxseed may diminish absorption of oral medications. Avoid administering flax at the same time as other medications, approximately 7 hours before or after.[4]

Interactions

None reported.

References

1. Fetrow CW, Avila J. *Professional's handbook of complementary and alternative medicines*. 3rd ed. Philadelphia (PA): Lippincott Williams & Wilkins; 2004:327–31.

2. Wynn SG, Marsden S. *Manual of natural veterinary medicine: science and tradition*. St. Louis (MO): Mosby; 2003:158.

3. Mills S, Bone K. *Principles and practice of phytotherapy: modern herbal medicine*. St. Louis (MO): Churchill Livingstone; 2000:54, 56, 157.

4. Wynn SG, Fougère B. *Veterinary herbal medicine*. St. Louis (MO): Elsevier; 2007:199, 301.

5. Broadfoot PJ, Palmquist RE, Jonston K, et al. *Integrating complementary medicine into veterinary practice*. Goldstein R, ed. Blackwell; 2008:708, 749. Available at: www.mediafire.com/?2s13ctmvv7tyb2k. Accessed January 15, 2012.

6. Pizzorno J, Murray M, Joiner-Bey H. *The clinician's handbook of natural medicine*. 2nd ed. St. Louis (MO): Churchill Livingstone; 2008:22, 47, 93–5, 350, 488, 716.

7. Stargrove M, Treasure J, McKee D. *Herb, nutrient, and drug interactions: clinical implications and therapeutic strategies*. St. Louis (MO): Mosby Elsevier; 2008:786.

Background

Garlic is one of the leading herbal supplements in humans,[1] and is available in various forms, including fresh raw or cooked garlic, garlic oil, dried powder, and aged garlic extract. The active ingredients in garlic include alliin and γ-glutamyl cysteine peptides. Alliin is converted by the enzyme allicinase (in the garlic) to allicin, which is an unstable product that rapidly degrades. The allicin is mainly responsible for garlic's pungent odor.[2,3]

Numerous scientific studies and clinical trials show a number of positive benefits of garlic. For example, garlic is used for cardiovascular disease,[4,5] for infectious diseases (broad-spectrum antibiotic and antifungal, antiviral, and antiparasitic activities),[5,6] as an antioxidant, and as an immunostimulating agent.[3] Garlic may lower serum cholesterol and lipids via inactivation of the enzyme hydroxymethylglutaryl coenzyme A (HGM-CoA) reductase, the same enzyme that is inhibited by cholesterol-lowering statin drugs.[3] Garlic exhibits antiplatelet activity,[7] although the risk of bleeding and interaction with antiplatelet or anticoagulant medications appears to be very low.[2]

Garlic may interact with various cytochrome P450 (CYP450) enzymes, which are involved in myriad metabolic pathways. Current evidence suggests that garlic inhibits CYP450 2E1, which is considered to be the main mechanism for garlic's hepatoprotective and chemoprotective properties.[3,8] Garlic may induce cell cycle arrest, inhibit inflammatory cytokines, inhibit P-glycoproteins (transporter proteins found in various tissues), and induce apoptosis in cancer cells.[3] Other mechanisms of garlic include a reduction in chemotherapy-induced mucositis (painful inflammation of the mucous membranes lining the gastrointestinal tract) associated with the chemotherapeutics methotrexate and 5-fluorouracil;[3] the ability to minimize cardiac arrhythmias, both ventricular and supraventricular;[6] a mild blood glucose–lowering effect; and the ability to protect against diabetes-induced side effects by inhibiting glycation.[9] Garlic may lower diastolic blood pressure and reduce heart rate,[4] inhibit angiogenesis,[7] and protect against *Helicobacter pylori*, which is the bacterium involved in gastric ulcer formation. Anecdotally, it was used topically in World War II to reduce infection.[8] Finally, garlic purportedly helps prevent stomach and/ or colorectal cancers. A direct toxic effect on sarcomas and gastric, colon, bladder, and prostate cancer cells was demonstrated in tissue culture. Garlic decreases nitrosamine and nitrite accumulation, and significantly prolongs survival time in mice injected with cancer cells.[8]

Different garlic preparations exhibit different constituent profiles and clinical effects.[6] Enteric-coated preparations release only a fraction of their allicin content and are not recommended.[3]

Indications
Suggested Uses in Humans
- Improves heart disease
- Supports patients with diabetes
- Controls hypercholesterolemia
- Inhibits cancer
- Fights *H. pylori* infection

Suggested Uses in Dogs and Cats
- Manages infections, including bacterial, fungal, and parasitic (internal and external)
- Inhibits cancer

Recommended Doses
In humans, the recommended dose for fresh garlic is 2.7–4 g/day. For the dried powder, the dose is 0.4–1.2 g/day, and the dose of garlic oil is 2–5 mg/day. The standard extract of garlic powder (Kwai) is dosed at 200–300 mg *q* 8 hr and the dose of aged garlic extract (Kyolic) is 300–800 mg *q* 8 hr. Other preparations are dosed based on the alliin concentration or the allicin-equivalent concentration. The desired alliin concentration is 4–12 mg/day and the allicin-equivalent concentration is dosed at 2–5 mg/day.[3] In dogs and cats, a variety of recommended doses appear in the veterinary and herbal literature. One reported dose is one clove of raw or cooked garlic/18.2 kg body weight/day.[4] In the author's experience, 1 clove of either raw or cooked garlic/9–22.7 kg body weight/ day (⅛–½ clove of garlic/4.5 kg cat or small dog/day) is an alternate dose. The dried herb can be administered at a dose of 15–20 mg/kg/ day (divided into three doses). Suggested ranges are 50–100 mg for

cats and small-breed dogs, 100–300 mg for medium-breed dogs, 300–600 mg for large-breed dogs, and 600–900 mg for giant-breed dogs.[6] A tincture (1:2 or 1:3) can be dosed at 0.5 mL/10 kg/day (divided into three doses).[6]

Side Effects

Garlic is generally considered a safe supplement when used at the proper dose. It is known that garlic can be toxic to dogs and particularly cats.[4] An overdose of garlic products in dogs and cats can cause oxidative injury to hemoglobin, resulting in methemoglobin formation and anemia, a low red blood cell count (because of the allicin content). The LD_{50} (the dose required to kill 50% of the test population) of allicin in mice is 120 mg/kg. The LD_{50} of garlic extracts in mice ranges from 0.5 mg/kg to >30 mL/kg. At the recommended doses listed above, garlic is unlikely to cause injury to dogs or cats. Pets known to be supplemented with garlic that experience decreases in red blood cell parameters on complete blood counts (eccentrocytosis appears to be a major diagnostic feature of garlic-induced hemolysis in dogs) should have their garlic dose adjusted accordingly and have their complete blood counts rechecked periodically to determine if garlic is the cause of the decreased red blood cell parameters.

In one study, four dogs administered 1.25 mL of garlic extract/kg body weight (5 g of whole garlic/kg) *q* 24 hr for 7 days experienced decreased erythrocyte counts, packed cell volumes, and hemoglobin concentrations 9–11 days following administration. Heinz body formation (red blood cells containing clumps of precipitated and denatured hemoglobin), an increase in erythrocyte-reduced glutathione concentration, and eccentrocytes (red blood cells with the hemoglobin shifted to the side) were also detected in these dogs. None of the dogs developed hemolytic anemia.[10]

Determining a "safe" dose of garlic is difficult. First, it is difficult to find a reported "safe" recommended dose in the literature, despite suggested doses by herbalists and veterinarians who recommend garlic. Second, many herbalists and naturopathic veterinarians use garlic in their patients at varying doses without obviously reported side effects. Third, many pet owners, often without the knowledge of their veterinarians, use fresh garlic or garlic supplements for their pets in varying amounts without obvious clinical signs prompting veterinary care. Because of the large number of pets receiving garlic products in some form without apparent side effects, it seems obvious that garlic may be used safely in pets.

Contraindications

None reported for humans; however, caution is advised in cats and small-breed dogs. Careful monitoring is recommended. Caution or avoidance is recommended in pets with anemia, and it is sometimes recommended to stop garlic or garlic supplements approximately 10 days before scheduled surgery (or to at least perform a complete blood count and, if needed, bleeding time).[3]

Interactions

Because of potential antiplatelet and/or anticoagulant effects (but despite the lack of clinical cases showing increased bleeding) garlic should be used carefully or avoided with anticoagulant medications (e.g., warfarin, aspirin) and herbs or supplements with similar activity (e.g., *Ginkgo biloba*, fish oil).[3,8] With careful monitoring, the use of garlic in patients being treated with anticoagulant or antiplatelet medications may result in a lowering of the dose of these medications. Garlic may also potentiate the effects of insulin or oral hypoglycemic agents,[4,6] and may exert a protective effect against the cardiotoxicity of doxorubicin and related anthracycline chemotherapy medications because of an antioxidant effect.[3] Garlic may allow for reduced doses of statin medications because of its ability to inactivate the enzyme HGM-CoA reductase.[3] Because of garlic's inhibition of one of the cytochrome enzymes (CYP450 2E1), elevated serum levels of medications that rely on this enzyme for metabolism may occur, such as acetaminophen.[3]

References

1. Packaged Facts. The U.S. herbal supplements market. 2001. Available at: http://www.packagedfacts.com/Herbal-Supplements-235863/. Accessed January 15, 2012.

2. Pizzorno J, Murray M. *Textbook of natural medicine*. 3rd ed. St. Louis (MO): Churchill Livingstone; 2005:726–34.

3. Stargrove M, Treasure J, McKee D. *Herb, nutrient, and drug interactions: clinical implications and therapeutic strategies.* St. Louis (MO): Mosby Elsevier; 2008:53–61.

4. Wynn SG, Marsden S. *Manual of natural veterinary medicine: science and tradition.* St. Louis (MO): Mosby; 2003:279.

5. Schoen A, Wynn SG. *Complementary and alternative veterinary medicine: principles and practice.* St. Louis (MO): Mosby; 1998:103, 315, 342–3, 368–9, 394.

6. Wynn S, Fougère B. *Veterinary herbal medicine.* St. Louis (MO): Elsevier; 2007:328–9, 555–8.

7. Broadfoot PJ, Palmquist RE, Jonston K, et al. *Integrating complementary medicine into veterinary practice.* Goldstein R, ed. Blackwell; 2008:654–5, 706. Available at: www.mediafire.com/?2s13ctmvv7tyb2k. Accessed January 15, 2012.

8. Fetrow CW, Avila J. *Professional's handbook of complementary and alternative medicines.* 3rd ed. Philadelphia (PA): Lippincott Williams & Wilkins; 2004:342–9.

9. Pizzorno J, Murray M, Joiner-Bey H. *The clinician's handbook of natural medicine.* 2nd ed. St. Louis (MO): Churchill Livingstone; 2008:218.

10. Lee KW, Yamato O, Tajima M, et al. Hematologic changes associated with the appearance of eccentrocytes after intragastric administration of garlic extract to dogs. *Am J Vet Res* 2000;61(11):1446–50.

GINGER

Background

Ginger, either the fresh or dried rhizome, is used as a nutritional (herbal) supplement. Ginger has potent anti-inflammatory effects via eicosanoid metabolism, has digestive and circulatory effects, and functions as an antioxidant with antineoplastic and antimicrobial properties.[1,2] The active ingredients in ginger are compounds called gingerols, as well as monoterpenes and sesquiterpenes.[1] Because of its anti-inflammatory effects, ginger is often used by patients with osteoarthritis—a painful, degenerative condition of joints—either by itself or in combination with nonsteroidal anti-inflammatory drugs (NSAIDs such as aspirin) or other anti-inflammatory herbs (e.g., garlic). Ginger inhibits the enzymes cyclo-oxygenase (COX) and lipoxygenase (LOX), enzymes that produce potent pro-inflammatory mediators, without producing side effects typically seen with COX or LOX inhibitors (e.g., ulcers).[3] In Chinese medicine, ginger has been used to stop bleeding in cases of "deficiency" or "cold"; however, as described below, there is some speculation that ginger consumption results in an increased risk of bleeding.[3] Ginger also exerts antinausea effects in patients treated with chemotherapy,[4] and may be helpful both before and after chemotherapy to reduce or prevent nausea in patients treated with cisplatin or other drugs that may induce vomiting.[5] This herb also has general antiemetic effects.[6] There is also some evidence supporting its use for treating heartworm in dogs.[7]

Indications

Suggested Uses in Humans

- Acts as an anti-inflammatory agent and controls pain
- Controls nausea
- Minimizes gastrointestinal ulcers

Suggested Uses in Dogs and Cats

- Acts as an anti-inflammatory agent and controls pain
- Controls nausea
- Minimizes gastrointestinal ulcers

Recommended Doses

Doses in humans range from 2 g/day to 4 g/day of either the fresh or dried rhizome or standardized extract. Alternatively, 1.25–3 mL of a tincture (1:5) can be administered q 8 hr or 0.25–0.75 mL of a fluid extract (1:1) q 8 hr.[3] Doses in dogs/cats/pets are extrapolated from doses used in people.

Side Effects

Ginger is considered a very safe herb and toxicity is minimal. Ginger is free of adverse effects at the recommended doses.[3]

Contraindications

Ginger may exhibit mild inhibitory effects on platelet aggregation, although *in vitro* studies are inconclusive and *in vivo* studies failed to consistently show definitive inhibition of platelet aggregation. At this time, no clear contraindications exist preventing the use of ginger in patients with hemostatic disorders or those taking anticoagulant or antiplatelet medications.[3]

Interactions

Despite the effects of ginger on COX and LOX inhibition, detectable clinical effects are unlikely and have not been reported. This suggests that ginger can be used safely with COX and LOX inhibitors, but monitoring the patient is prudent. Because of the antinausea/antiemetic effects of ginger, patients can be administered garlic with medications such as certain chemotherapeutic agents (e.g., cisplatin) or general anesthetics that can cause nausea. Ginger has been used in Chinese medicine to stop bleeding. At recommended doses, ginger presents no significant risk of bleeding in patients taking oral vitamin K antagonists or antiplatelet medications, but patient monitoring is encouraged if these drugs are coadministered with ginger. Finally, there is some evidence to suggest that when coadministered with nonsteroidal anti-inflammatory drugs, ginger has an additive effect, and can benefit patients with osteoarthritis.[3]

References

1. Fetrow CW, Avila J. *Professional's handbook of complementary and alternative medicines.* 3rd ed. Philadelphia (PA): Lippincott Williams & Wilkins; 2004:352–8.

2. Mills S, Bone K. *Principles and practice of phytotherapy: modern herbal medicine.* St. Louis (MO): Churchill Livingstone; 2000:394–402.

3. Stargrove M, Treasure J, McKee D. *Herb, nutrient, and drug interactions: clinical implications and therapeutic strategies.* St. Louis (MO): Mosby Elsevier; 2008:62–9.

4. Wynn S, Marsden S. *Manual of natural veterinary medicine: science and tradition.* St. Louis (MO): Mosby; 2003.

5. Pizzorno J, Murray M, Joiner-Bey H. *The clinician's handbook of natural medicine.* 2nd ed. St. Louis (MO): Churchill Livingstone; 2008:535, 537.

6. Broadfoot PJ, Palmquist RE, Jonston K, et al. *Integrating complementary medicine into veterinary practice.* Goldstein R, ed. Blackwell; 2008:302, 313. Available at: www.mediafire.com/?2s13ctmvv7tyb2k. Accessed January 15, 2012.

7. Merawin LT, Arifah AK, Sani RA, et al. Screening of microfilaricidal effects of plant extracts against *Dirofilaria immitis. Res Vet Sci* 2010;88(1):142–7.

(*GINKGO BILOBA*)

Background

The ginkgo leaf is used as a nutritional supplement as the active constituents include terpenes (ginkgolides) and flavonoids.[1] Most of the clinical research has used concentrated standardized extracts; however, the whole-leaf dry extracts or liquid extracts of the whole leaf are often used in clinical practice.[2]

Ginkgo leaf extract has been used in patients with Alzheimer's disease and other forms of dementia because it increases cerebral blood flow.[3,4] Ginkgo, however, has not shown any benefit in enhancing memory in normal healthy adults with intact cognition.[5] Ginkgo increases cerebral blood flow and tissue perfusion as a result of arterial vasodilation,[1] and ginkgolide B inhibits platelet aggregation and inhibits platelet-activating factor (PAF).[2,3] Other benefits of ginkgo include antioxidant properites[2] and chemoprotective, neuroprotective, and anti-ischemic effects.[5]

Indications

Suggested Uses in Humans
- Improves Alzheimer's disease/dementias

Suggested Uses in Dogs and Cats
- Supports patients with cognitive disorders
- Controls feline asthma patients
- Helps patients with heart failure[2]

Recommended Doses

In humans, 3–8 mL/day of a 1:1 fluid extract or 120–240 mg/day in divided doses (*q* 8–12 hr) of a standardized dry whole-leaf extract are recommended.[6] In dogs and cats, recommended doses are 25–300 mg/kg *q* 8 hr of a powder or capsule; 0.5–1 mL/10 kg *q* 8 hr of a 1:2–1:3 tincture; and 10–50 mg/10 kg *q* 8–12 hr of a standardized extract (50:1).[3] In the author's experience, an alternative dosing regimen is a 100 mg capsule/11.4 kg dog or 4.5 kg cat *q* 8–12 hr; and ¼–½ teaspoon of powder/11.4 kg dog or 4.5 kg cat *q* 8–12 hr; and 5–10 drops of a 1:5 tincture/4.5–9 kg dog or 4.5 kg cat *q* 8–12 hr.

Side Effects

Ginkgo is considered a safe herb with an excellent safety profile. However, there are safety concerns because of the potential for increased bleeding, especially subdural hematomas and seizures, if large amounts of ginkgo seeds are consumed.[3]

Contraindications

None reported.

Interactions

In vitro, ginkgo extracts show platelet inhibition.[7] Clinically, there are no reliable reports of spontaneous bleeding as a result of ginkgo administration by itself. However, individual patient assessment is warranted when prescribing ginkgo to patients prescribed other medications or other supplements (e.g., high-dose fish oil, garlic, ginseng) that may possess anticoagulant/antiplatelet properties. In the author's experience, because ginkgo may exert protective effects on the gastrointestinal system against the formation of ulcers, ginkgo may be a better choice than other medications (e.g., aspirin) when mild anticoagulation is needed. Additionally, the use of ginkgo might permit a reduction in other anticoagulants.[6] Ginkgo extracts may shorten the duration of anesthesia. It is therefore advised to refrain from supplementing pets with ginkgo for approximately 10 days prior to anesthesia/surgery, if possible.[6] Ginkgo may reduce cyclosporine- and aminoglycoside-induced nephrotoxicity, as well as the ototoxicity associated with aminoglycoside administration and the cardiotoxicity that may be seen with doxorubicin or other anthracycline chemotherapy medications.[6] Supplementation with ginkgo may increase blood pressure if administered concurrently with thiazide diuretics.[6,7]

References

1. Broadfoot PJ, Palmquist RE, Jonston K, et al. *Integrating complementary medicine into veterinary practice.* Goldstein R, ed. Blackwell; 2008:654–5, 707. Available at: www.mediafire.com/?2s13ctmvv7tyb2k. Accessed January 15, 2012.

2. Wynn SG, Marsden S. *Manual of natural veterinary medicine: science and tradition.* St. Louis (MO): Mosby; 2003:58, 78, 244–5, 533.

3. Wynn SG, Fougère B. *Veterinary herbal medicine.* Mosby Elsevier; 2007:300, 356, 562–4.

4. Pizzorno J, Murray M, Joiner-Bey H. *The clinician's handbook of natural medicine.* 2nd ed. St. Louis (MO): Churchill Livingstone; 2008:45–7.

5. Mills S, Bone K. *Principles and practice of phytotherapy: modern herbal medicine.* St. Louis (MO): Churchill Livingstone; 2000:90, 119, 197, 404–15.

6. Stargrove M, Treasure J, McKee D. *Herb, nutrient, and drug interactions: clinical implications and therapeutic strategies.* St. Louis (MO): Mosby Elsevier; 2008:69–79.

7. Fetrow CW, Avila J. *Professional's handbook of complementary and alternative medicines.* 3rd ed. Philadelphia (PA): Lippincott Williams & Wilkins; 2004:358–65.

(*PANAX GINSENG*)

Background

Ginseng is an herb commonly used in traditional Chinese medicine. Confusion has existed regarding what constitutes "ginseng" because of the different species of plants that are called ginseng. Currently, *Panax ginseng* is the genus and species of plant used synonymously with ginseng (the pharmacopoeial name is *Radix ginseng*). Common names for this plant include ginseng, Korean ginseng, Chinese ginseng, Asian ginseng, and Oriental ginseng. American ginseng (also called wild American ginseng) is *Panax quinquefolius*. Siberian ginseng is a different plant that currently goes by the name eleuthero (*Eleutherococcus senticosus*). White ginseng (*Ren shen*) is the dried peeled root, whereas red ginseng (*Hong shen*, considered warmer and stronger or more *Yang* than white ginseng) is the root steamed before drying.[1]

The active ingredients in ginseng are steroid saponins called ginsenosides. More than 30 ginsenosides have been identified to date, which make up approximately 3% of the herb.[1]

Ginseng is unique among herbs because it is considered an adaptogen. By definition, adaptogens are nonspecific and nontoxic, normalize homeostasis, and help the patient adapt to various stressors.[1] Ginseng has a wide range of actions, including immunomodulation, antineoplastic properties,[2] neuroendocrine effects, and positive effects on cognitive, athletic, and sexual performance.[3] Ginseng can be used in almost any patient as an aid to adapt to any type of stress/illness.[4] Ginseng enhances cell-mediated immunity (one of the main branches of the immune system), especially natural killer (NK) cell activity.[3] This makes ginseng useful anytime enhanced immune activity (e.g., infections, neoplasia, etc.) is required. Ginseng may increase the effectiveness of some vaccines, possibly from enhanced antigen presenting cell (APC) activity, although the clinical significance remains to be established.[1] Ginseng may also be beneficial to cancer patients by inducing cellular differentiation and by an antimutagenic effect.[3] In addition, ginseng is beneficial in reducing toxicity from both chemotherapy (probably from protecting against leukopenia, reducing actual chemical toxicity, and enhancing stress resistance) and radiation therapy.[3]

It is important for consumers to note that there is often variable quality and composition of commercial products claiming to contain ginseng. Adulteration with contaminating species (such as *Periploca sepium*, a cardiotoxic herb) has been identified, especially in supplements imported from China.[1]

Indications

Suggested Uses in Humans

- Helps people adapt to stress/illness
- Enhances stamina
- Increases mental alertness/cognitive performance
- Serves as an adjunct to radiation/chemotherapy
- Acts as an immunoprotective agent/immunomodulator

Suggested Uses in Dogs and Cats

- Helps animals adapt to stress/illness
- Serves as an adjunct to radiation/chemotherapy
- Acts as an immunoprotective agent/immunomodulator

Recommended Doses

In humans, 3 mL/day of a 1:1 fluid extract, 2–10 g/day (divided and administered *q* 8–12 hr) of the dried root, and 100 mg of a 5:1 4% ginsenoside solid extract *q* 12 hr are recommended doses.[1] In dogs and cats, a recommended dose is 250–500 mg/kg.[2] In the author's experience, an alternative dose is one 100 mg capsule/11.4 kg dog or 4.5 kg cat *q* 8–12 hr, 1.25–2.5 mL (¼–½ teaspoon of powder)/11.4 kg dog or 4.5 kg cat *q* 8–12 hr, 5–10 drops of a 1:5 tincture/4.5–9 kg dog or 4.5 kg cat *q* 8–12 hr, or 1–2 drops/0.45–0.9 kg *q* 8–12 hr.

Side Effects

Ginseng is among the safest herbs used in natural medicine. Toxicity is minimal and the herbs are free of adverse effects at the recommended doses. Isolated case reports of people taking "ginseng" and experiencing adverse effects while taking other medications (such as warfarin or digitalis glycosides) do exist; however, these case reports are problematic because the exact species of the plant that constitutes "ginseng" in the actual herbal formula ingested is often not clear.

Contraindications

None reported.

Interactions

Experimental evidence suggests a modulating effect of ginseng on P-glycoprotein, a transporter protein involved in phase III drug metabolism. The mechanisms of drug resistance modulation or pump-mediated interactions between ginseng and conventional medications have not been fully explained.[1] Doxorubicin cardiotoxicity may be reduced when coadministered with ginseng, and intestinal bacteria may hydrolyze ginseng into novel metabolites that possess antineoplastic activity.[1] A synergistic effect between amoxicillin and related beta-lactam antibiotics administered with ginseng results in increased antibacterial effect.[1]

When administered with chemotherapy agents (particularly antitumor antibiotics and platinum medications), ginseng may act as a chemosensitizer as well as a protector against drug toxicities. Proposed mechanisms of action include multidrug resistance disabling, potentiation of cytotoxic activity, protection of healthy cells, and enhancement of the immune system during myelosuppression (suppression of bone marrow).[1] Ginseng may interfere with the analgesic effects of morphine and related medications and may inhibit the uptake of the neurotransmitters glutamate, dopamine, norepinephrine, serotonin, and γ-aminobutyric acid (GABA) in a dose-dependent fashion. Care should be exercised when combining monoamine oxidase (MAO) inhibitors with ginseng.[1]

References

1. Stargrove M, Treasure J, McKee D. *Herb, nutrient, and drug interactions: clinical implications and therapeutic strategies.* St. Louis (MO): Mosby Elsevier; 2008:80–7.

2. Wynn SG, Fougère B. *Veterinary herbal medicine.* St. Louis (MO): Mosby Elsevier; 2007:303, 332–3, 351–3.

3. Mills S, Bone K. *Principles and practice of phytotherapy: modern herbal medicine.* St. Louis (MO): Churchill Livingstone; 2000:418–30, 538.

4. Pizzorno J, Murray M. *Textbook of natural medicine.* 3rd ed. St. Louis (MO): Churchill Livingstone; 2005:707, 923.

GLUCOSAMINE

(GLUCOSAMINE SULFATE GLUCOSAMINE HYDROCHLORIDE, N-ACETYL-D-GLUCOSAMINE)

Background

Glucosamine is an aminosugar (a molecule that contains a sugar as well as nitrogen) made from glucose that is incorporated into articular cartilage. Glucosamine is the most common chondroprotective (joint-protecting) supplement used in patients either diagnosed or suspected of having osteoarthritis—the painful degeneration of the articular cartilage that lines the ends of long bones. Glucosamine can be synthesized in the body, but significant amounts of glucosamine are not normally found in most diets. Glucosamine supplements are derived from the exoskeletons of shrimp, lobsters, and crab.[1] Glucosamine is available in three forms: glucosamine sulfate, glucosamine hydrochloride, and N-acetyl-D-glucosamine. All three forms of glucosamine may be effective; however, glucosamine sulfate is the form most commonly used in research and therefore probably the preferred form. It is speculated that the sulfur portion of glucosamine sulfate, rather than the glucosamine portion, may be more important for joint health and may be an important reason why glucosamine sulfate supplements appear to be effective in helping pets with arthritis.[2]

Glucosamine activates chondrocytes (cartilage cells) via modulation of the pro-inflammatory mediator interleukin-1 (IL-1), and stimulates the production of various components of cartilage such as proteoglycans, polysulfated glycosaminoglycans, and collagen.[2,3] Glucosamine sulfate increases serum sulfur concentrations, which further allows the production of cartilage, as well as inhibiting several enzymes that destroy cartilage, such as serine proteases, collagnease, superoxide radicals, and phospholipase A2.[2] Glucosamine sulfate exerts an anti-inflammatory effect by a mechanism different from inhibition of prostaglandin synthesis, most likely by inhibition of the nuclear factor kappa B pathway.[2]

A number of studies in humans and animals show that glucosamine is as effective as nonsteroidal anti-inflammatory drugs (NSAIDs, e.g., aspirin-related drugs) for patients with osteoarthritis. In addition, glucosamine sulfate is free of the potentially serious side effects that can occur with NSAID administration, such as gastric ulcers and kidney damage.[4,5] Nonetheless, there are some reports that question the effectiveness of glucosamine for relieving joint pain. Careful evaluation of those negative reports indicated that many of the participants were permitted to take acetaminophen along with the glucosamine. It was proposed that acetaminophen in some way interfered with the participants receiving the full benefit of the glucosamine supplement. It is also potentially likely that study design or some other factors resulted in a lack of perceived benefit to glucosamine supplementation. To date, research, including clinical studies and clinical experience from myriad people and pets using glucosamine supplements, support the efficacy of the supplements in relieving pain, inflammation, and helping to rebuild damaged cartilage.[6]

Indications

Suggested Uses in Humans
- Supports patients with osteoarthritis

Suggested Uses in Dogs and Cats
- Supports patients with osteoarthritis
- Helps feline patients with bladder diseases such as feline lower urinary tract disease (FLUTD) and chronic cystitis

Recommended Doses

The typical dose in humans is 500 mg q 8 hr. For acute pain and injury and to accelerate tissue repair, initial doses of 3,000–4,500 mg/day for 3–5 days are often recommended.[2] In dogs and cats, recommended doses vary depending on the product. As a guideline, a starting dose of 250–1,500 mg/day (in divided doses) is recommended.[4] In the author's experience, an alternative starting dose of 20–100 mg/kg q 12 hr is appropriate. Typical doses of products developed for pets are 1,000–1,500 mg of glucosamine/day for a 22.7–45.5 kg dog and 250–500 mg/day for smaller dogs and cats. Doses of joint supplements are typically reduced after 4–8 weeks once clinical signs improve or resolve, to help minimize costs.

Side Effects

Glucosamine is very safe. Mild gastrointestinal upset is rarely observed, which may be avoided by taking glucosamine with food.[2] There have been some concerns about using glucosamine supplements (glucosamine is made from glucose) in patients with diabetes mellitus. Studies in humans demonstrate that supplementation with glucosamine at recommended doses does not interact adversely with insulin or oral hypoglycemic medications, or result in significant alterations in glucose metabolism.[2,7]

Contraindications

Glucosamine may be contraindicated in people or pets with allergies to shellfish.[2]

Interactions

Human patients prescribed diuretics may require higher doses of glucosamine supplements to obtain the full therapeutic benefits. This is likely also true in pets. Additionally, because glucosamine sulfate is stabilized with a mineral salt (sodium chloride or potassium chloride) electrolyte alterations may occur in patients taking both diuretics and glucosamine. Such patients should be monitored for electrolyte imbalances.[2] Acetaminophen may interfere with the actions of glucosamine sulfate because of consumption of the sulfate provided by glucosamine sulfate during sulfate metabolism of the acetaminophen.[2] A synergistic effect between glucosamine sulfate and NSAIDs may allow for a reduction in NSAID dose in patients with osteoarthritis.[2] Glucosamine joint supplements often contain other potentially synergistic ingredients, including vitamin C, manganese, chondroitin sulfate, and methylsulfonylmethane (MSM). These combinations are safe and effective and may be more effective than supplements containing only glucosamine sulfate. More research is needed to address this issue.[2] Finally, oligomeric proanthocyanidins (OPCs), which are plant secondary metabolites (most widely provided by grapeseed extract and pine bark extract), bind to collagen and elastin. These compounds reportedly protect collagen and elastin from the degradative enzymes collagenases and elastinases, respectively, generated during inflammatory. As a result they may have a synergistic effect with supplements containing these OPCs with glucosamine sulfate.[2]

References

1. Pizzorno J, Murray M. *Textbook of natural medicine*. 3rd ed. St. Louis (MO): Churchill Livingstone; 2005:987–91.

2. Stargrove M, Treasure J, McKee D. *Herb, nutrient, and drug interactions: clinical implications and therapeutic strategies*. St. Louis (MO): Mosby Elsevier; 2008:757–63.

3. Wynn SG, Marsden S. *Manual of natural veterinary medicine: science and tradition*. St. Louis (MO): Mosby; 2003:368–9, 447–8.

4. Schoen A, Wynn SG. *Complementary and alternative veterinary medicine: principles and practice*. St. Louis (MO): Mosby; 1998:54–7, 64–5.

5. Broadfoot PJ, Palmquist RE, Jonston K, et al. *Integrating complementary medicine into veterinary practice*. Goldstein R, ed. Blackwell; 2008:21, 132, 424, 434. Available at: www.mediafire.com/?2s13ctmvv7tyb2k. Accessed January 15, 2012.

6. Pizzorno J, Murray M, Joiner-Bey H. *The clinician's handbook of natural medicine*. 2nd ed. St. Louis (MO): Churchill Livingstone; 2008:558, 563.

7. Simon RR, Marks V, Leeds AR, et al. A comprehensive review of oral glucosamine use and effects on glucose metabolism in normal and diabetic individuals. *Diabetes Metab Res Rev* 2011;27(1):14–27. Available at: http://www.ncbi.nlm.nih.gov/pmc/articles/PMC3042150/pdf/dmrr0027-0014.pdf. Accessed February 20, 2012.

(L-GLUTAMINE)

Background

Glutamine is the most abundant amino acid in blood and muscle and is a preferred energy source for rapidly dividing cells, especially those lining the gastrointestinal tract (enterocytes).[1] Glutamine serves as an intermediary for gluconeogenesis (the production of glucose from amino acids to provide energy) from amino acids that are released by skeletal muscles during stress.[1]

Glutamine is available either in the diet or through supplementation and is made by the body from glutamate and ammonia. Food sources include animal and plant proteins (e.g., meat, fish, dairy products, cabbage, legumes).[1] Supplementation may be necessary because of increased needs by the body and during times of stress, such as illness and exercise.[1] Although the terms "glutamine" and "L-glutamine" (one of the two forms or "isomers" of glutamine) are used interchangeably, the other isomer, D-glutamine, possesses no biologic activity.[1]

Glutamine stimulates intestinal mucosal growth, decreases mucosal atrophy,[2] serves as a fuel source for enteroctyes, decreases bacterial and toxin translocation across the intestinal mucosa or lining (i.e., decreases "leaky gut syndrome"), plays a role in acid-base balance by removing ammonia from the blood, regenerates glutathione,[2] decreases muscle protein loss, modulates the immune system by enhancing interleukin-6 (IL-6) levels and lymphocyte (a particular type of infection-fighting white blood cell) function,[1] and is used to improve/limit cachexia.[3] Glutamine has anabolic effects on skeletal muscle and may therefore be helpful in the form of supplementation as part of an exercise regimen.[1] An oral rinse containing glutamine purportedly reduces stomatitis (inflammation of membranes in the mouth, including gums, tongue, cheeks, etc.) associated with chemotherapy.[2,3,4]

Indications

Suggested Uses in Humans

- Helps gastrointestinal diseases
- Minimizes side effects (e.g., stomatitis, mucositis, gastroenteritis) associated with chemotherapy and radiation therapy

- Minimizes/improves cachexia
- Supports patients with severe illnesses such as infection with HIV, sepsis, cardiac diseases
- Supplements individuals during exercise/weight lifting
- Helps trauma patients
- Improves severe burns

Suggested Uses in Dogs and Cats
- Helps gastrointestinal diseases
- Minimizes side effects (e.g., stomatitis, mucositis, gastroenteritis) associated with chemotherapy and radiation therapy
- Supports patients with critical illnesses
- Helps trauma patients
- Supplements elite athletes

Recommended Doses

In humans, the usual dose is 100 mg *q* 8 hr; however, doses up to 30 g *q* 24 hr have been used in patients with severe illness.[1] In dogs and cats, the typical dose is 250–3,000 mg/day (divided).[3]

Side Effects

Glutamine is very safe, even at high doses.

Contraindications

Many anticonvulsant medications block glutamate activity in the brain. Because glutamine can be converted to glutamate, caution should be used when supplementing patients with glutamine, especially at high doses, concurrently with anticonvulsant medications.[1] There are some data indicating increased glutamine levels in certain brain diseses,[5] and excessive glutamate may serve as a stimulus for the growth of malignant brain tumors. Additionally, cancer cells use glutamine to grow and metastasize *in vitro*.[2] Until more information is available, patients with nerve-damaging, chronic neurological diseases (e.g., multiple sclerosis or recent neurological surgeries, such as for brain tumors) are encouraged to limit their intake of supplemental glutamine to approximately 5–10 g/day.[5]

Interactions

None reported.

References

1. Pizzorno J, Murray M. *Textbook of natural medicine.* 3rd ed. St. Louis (MO): Churchill Livingstone; 2005:993–9.

2. Wynn SG, Marsden S. *Manual of natural veterinary medicine: science and tradition.* St. Louis (MO): Mosby; 2003:163, 204, 190, 194, 204, 399.

3. Schoen A, Wynn SG. *Complementary and alternative veterinary medicine: principles and practice.* St. Louis (MO): Mosby; 1998:98, 102.

4. Broadfoot PJ, Palmquist RE, Jonston K, et al. *Integrating complementary medicine into veterinary practice.* Goldstein R, ed. Blackwell; 2008:301, 323, 339, 722, 735. Available at: www.mediafire.com/?2s13ctmvv7tyb2k. Accessed January 15, 2012.

5. Dharmananda S. Amino acid supplements 1: glutamine. With reference to the Related Compound Glutamate. Available at: http://www.itmonline.org/arts /glutamine.htm. Accessed March 13, 2012.

(*CAMELLIA SINENSIS*)

Background

Green tea (young leaves, leaf buds, and tips) is a commonly used supplement for its antioxidant and anticancer properties.[1] "Medicinal" green tea is stabilized, dried immediately after harvesting, and rolled, which means the crude herb is approximately equivalent to its natural state at the time of harvesting.[2] Green tea includes various flavonoids, vitamins, minerals, amino acids, caffeine, and polyphenols (a type of antioxidant). The four principal polyphenolic compounds in green tea are called catechins (epicatechin [EC], epigallocatechin [EGC], epicatechin gallate [ECG], and the principal compound epigallocatechin gallate [EGCG]), which are responsible for most of the observed beneficial clinical effects.[2] In contrast, black tea is dried after being rolled, which allows oxidative enzymatic changes to take place. These changes result in the formation of red-brown theaflavins, thearubigins, and polymeric tannins, which are all absent from green tea.[2]

Although people often drink green tea for its health benefits, extremely high volumes are required because of the poor oral bioavailability of the active polyphenols. Approximately 10 cups of green tea/person/day would be necessary to begin to approach the therapeutic dose. Therefore, the supplemental form of green tea is usually consumed for health benefits.[2]

EGCG promotes cancer cell apoptosis (programmed cell death) and inhibits angiogenesis (formation of new blood vessels) by interfering with vascular endothelial growth factor (VEGF) function.[2,3] EGCG exhibits synergistic effects with chemotherapeutics and modifies drug resistance (through inhibition of P-glycoprotein, a transported protein involved in drug metabolism).[2] EGCG inhibits receptor tyrosine kinase activity, and may reduce secondary tumors caused by cisplatin usage.[2] Green tea also exhibits anti-inflammatory and antibacterial (e.g., against various bacteria, including methicillin-resistant *Staphylococcus aureus*) activities.[4] Finally, green tea may reduce cholesterol, abrogates atherosclerosis, exhibits antiplatelet effects, decreases the formation of dental caries, and inhibits tumor metastasis (distant spread).[3–5]

Indications

Suggested Uses in Humans

- Functions as an antioxidant
- Benefits cancer patients
- Helps patients with atopic dermatitis

Suggested Uses in Dogs and Cats

- Functions as an antioxidant
- Benefits cancer patients

Recommended Doses

In humans, traditional Chinese medicine guidelines recommend 4–12 g of dried powder/day (divided).[2] Approximately 300–750 mg of polyphenols/dose is recommended.[2,5] Green tea extracts are often standardized to 60% polyphenols and contain 1–4% caffeine. In dogs and cats, 10–20 mg/kg *q* 12 hr of a standardized 34% EGCG product is suggested.[6]

Side Effects

Green tea is a very safe supplement with no reported side effects.

Contraindications

None reported.

Interactions

Administering green tea with topical corticosteroids can improve response in refractory atopic dermatitis, which permits a reduced dose of corticosteroids (and a concomitant decrease in possible side effects associated with corticosteroid use).[2] EGCG may reduce doxorubicin-induced cardiomyopathy and increases cancer cell sensitivity by inhibiting P-glycoprotein.[2] EGCG functions synergistically with beta-lactam antibiotics (e.g., penicillin, etc.) and can reverse beta-lactam antibiotic resistance by modulating the bacterial phenotype in methicillin-resistant strains of *Staphylococcus aureus*.[2] Tamoxifen-induced (a chemotherapeutic) apoptosis is increased by EGCG *in vitro*.[2] Historically, there has been a concern that green tea might antagonize anticoagulant drugs such as warfarin. There are currently no credible reports supporting this speculation; however, the current practice is to avoid excessive tea consumption in patients using oral anticoagulants and antithrombotic medications.[2]

References

1. Schoen A, Wynn SG. *Complementary and alternative veterinary medicine: principles and practice.* St. Louis (MO): Mosby; 1998:103.

2. Stargrove M, Treasure J, McKee D. *Herb, nutrient, and drug interactions: clinical implications and therapeutic strategies.* St. Louis (MO): Mosby Elsevier; 2008:91–8.

3. Broadfoot PJ, Palmquist RE, Jonston K, et al. *Integrating complementary medicine into veterinary practice.* Goldstein R, ed. Blackwell; 2008:660, 706, 710. Available at: www.mediafire.com/?2s13ctmvv7tyb2k. Accessed January 15, 2012.

4. Fetrow CW, Avila J. *Professional's handbook of complementary and alternative medicines.* 3rd ed. Philadelphia (PA): Lippincott Williams & Wilkins; 2004:398–402.

5. Pizzorno J, Murray M. *Textbook of natural medicine.* 3rd ed. St. Louis (MO): Churchill Livingstone; 2005:800.

6. Wynn SG, Marsden S. *Manual of natural veterinary medicine: science and tradition.* St. Louis (MO): Mosby; 2003:401.

HAWTHORN

(*CRATAEGUS LAEVIGATA, C. MONOGYNA, C. OXYACANTHA*)

Background

Hawthorn is an herb well-known for its use in the treatment of heart disease because of the flavonoid and oligomeric proanthocyanidin (OPC) content.[1] Typically the leaves and flowers are used, although traditionally fruits and berries have also been used.[1] Hawthorn exhibits several clinically beneficial effects on the heart, including antiarrhythmic properties (to maintain a normal heart rhythm), positive inotropic effects (to increase force of contraction), increased coronary blood flow, decreased myocardial energy utilization, decreased atrio-ventricular conduction time, and decreased cardiac excitability.[1-5] Hawthorn inhibits the enzyme phosphodiesterase,[6] increases nitric oxide–mediated endothelial relaxation (causing dilation of blood vessels), inhibits platelet aggregation, inhibits phospholipase A2, exhibits antioxidant properties, exhibits hypolipidemic (lipid-lowering) properties, acts similarly to angiotensin-1-converting enzyme (ACE) inhibitors to help regulate blood pressure, and increases the duration of cardiac muscle action potential by blocking potassium channels.[1,7]

Indications

Suggested Uses in Humans
- Improves heart disease
- Supports cancer patients during chemotherapy

Suggested Uses in Dogs and Cats
- Improves heart disease
- Supports cancer patients during chemotherapy

Recommended Doses

In humans, the dried leaf and flower is administered at a dose of 1,500 mg *q* 6–8 hr. The tincture is dosed at 3–7 mL *q* 12–24 hr, and the dose of the standardized extract (2.2% flavonoids or 18.75% OPC) is 600–900 mg *q* 8–24 hr.[7] In dogs and cats, 25–300 mg/kg/ day (divided doses) is recommended.[1]

Side Effects

Hawthorne is considered a very safe supplement in both people and pets.

Contraindications

None reported. Avoid administering hawthorn to patients allergic to the plant.[8]

Interactions

Because of similarities between hawthorn and digitalis-type cardiac glycosides (which stimulate the heart muscle), there is the potential to cause adverse reactions when both hawthorn and digitalis glycosides are coadministered.[2,8] However, this interaction has not been observed clinically.[7] Further, combining hawthorn with digitalis glycosides may permit a lower dose of the digitalis glycosides because of the additive positive inotropic effects.[3] To date, hawthorn has not been shown to interact negatively or cause any adverse effects when prescribed with any other cardiac medications.[7] Hawthorn may reduce the cardiotoxicity seen with doxorubicin and other anthracycline chemotherapeutic agents.[7] Combining hawthorn with diuretics in patients with congestive heart failure may lead to further reduction of symptoms and reduced adverse effects associated with diruetics.[7]

References

1. Wynn SG, Fougère B. *Veterinary herbal medicine*. St. Louis (MO): Mosby Elsevier; 2007:311, 579–81.

2. Schoen A, Wynn SG. *Complementary and alternative veterinary medicine: principles and practice*. St. Louis (MO): Mosby; 1998:318, 347–8.

3. Wynn SG, Marsden S. *Manual of natural veterinary medicine: science and tradition*. St. Louis (MO): Mosby; 2003:77, 90.

4. Broadfoot PJ, Palmquist RE, Jonston K, et al. *Integrating complementary medicine into veterinary practice*. Goldstein R, ed. Blackwell; 2008:653–4. Available at: www.mediafire.com/?2s13ctmvv7tyb2k. Accessed January 15, 2012.

5. Pizzorno J, Murray M, Joiner-Bey H. *The clinician's handbook of natural medicine*. 2nd ed. St. Louis (MO): Churchill Livingstone; 2008:53–5.

6. Mills S, Bone K. *Principles and practice of phytotherapy: modern herbal medicine*. St. Louis (MO): Churchill Livingstone; 2000:439–46.

7. Stargrove M, Treasure J, McKee D. *Herb, nutrient, and drug interactions: clinical implications and therapeutic strategies*. St. Louis (MO): Mosby Elsevier; 2008:99–103.

8. Fetrow CW, Avila J. *Professional's handbook of complementary and alternative medicines*. 3rd ed. Philadelphia (PA): Lippincott Williams & Wilkins; 2004:414–16.

Background

Hyaluronic acid (HA) is a high-molecular-weight glycosaminoglycan composed of long chains of glucuronic acid and N-acetyl-glucosamine.[1] HA is commonly used as a joint supplement extracted from rooster combs or bovine tracheas, or (more commonly) generated using a patented process by fermentation using nonpathogenic *Streptococcus* spp.[2,3] These organisms produce an outer coating of hyaluronic acid that is sloughed off in the media and then purified. An approved preservative is required or the bacteria will degrade the HA, making it pro-inflammatory. Approved preservatives (by the U.S. Food and Drug Administration, FDA) that are safe to include in HA products include 1,2-propanediol, methyl paraben, and propyl paraben. Commercial HA products may also contain other preservatives/ingredients, including vitamin C; ethylenediaminetetraacetic acid (EDTA); potassium or sodium sorbate; potassium, sodium, or calcium citrate; grapeseed extract; tea tree extract; and citric acid. These ingredients on their own do not adequately stabilize the HA. Adding stabilizers such as xantham gum, carbopol, or guar gum increases the viscosity so that the HA degradation cannot be detected (when HA degrades, it becomes thinner).

The concentration of HA in nutritional supplements should be 1% (10 mg/mL), which is the highest concentration of high-molecular-weight HA that can be put into solution. Products that claim to have a higher concentration use low-molecular-weight HA (often <200,000 daltons), which is pro-inflammatory, not anti-inflammatory.[4]

The proposed mechanisms of action of HA include reduced swelling at the site of injury by decreasing white blood cell migration and infiltration into the affected tissue (via binding to the CD44 binding site on white blood cells), decreasing the number of white blood cells at the site of trauma (resulting in reduced swelling and pain), inhibiting the arachidonic acid pathway, and blocking serine protease (enzyme) activity so that lysyl bradykinin, bradykinin, and arachidonic acid cannot be produced (resulting in decreased pain).[4,5] HA inhibits the formation of pro-inflammatory interleukins (IL-4 and IL-6) as well as tumor necrosis factor (TNF), blocking both acute and chronic inflammation.[4] Clinically, HA has been used to improve joint fluid in arthritis, as a surgical aid in eye surgery, and to facilitate the healing and regeneration of surgical wounds.[6] It has also been used in various skin diseases such as actinic keratitis and to improve wound healing (e.g., diabetic ulcers, skin inflammation from radiation treatments).[7] Finally, HA is involved in embryogenesis, metastasis, tumor progression, and tissue turnover.[8]

Indications
Suggested Uses in Humans
- Improves osteoarthritis, bursitis, muscle soreness, fibromyalgia
- Improves skin tone and suppleness, reduces wrinkling/aging of skin, minimizes sunburns, helps with wound healing and healing postsurgically
- Slows hair loss (HA appears to thicken hair and/or result in hair growth)
- Normalizes elevated liver enzymes
- Reduces plaque on teeth
- Controls postsurgical pain
- Assists during cataract surgery
- Supports patients with heart disease
- Supports patients with cancer
- Helps patients with Alzheimer's disease

Suggested Uses in Dogs and Cats
- Improves osteoarthritis
- Normalizes elevated liver enzymes
- Helps control Cushing's and Addison's disease

Recommended Doses
An anecdotal dose in humans is 50 mg (1 teaspoon of a 1% solution) q 8–12 hr. No specific recommendations in dogs and cats appear to have been established.

Side Effects
None reported.

Contraindications

None reported, except that some cats have shown sensitivity to 1,2-propanediol, which is also called propylene glycol (one of the FDA-approved preservatives used in HA supplements). Feline products should have a reduced concentration of this preservative.

Interactions

None reported.

References

1. Strauss EJ, Hart JA, Miller MD, et al. Hyaluronic acid viscosupplementation and osteoarthritis: current uses and future directions. *Am J Sports Med* 2009;37(8):1636–44.

2. Kalman DS, Heimer M, Valdeon A, et al. Effect of a natural extract of chicken combs with a high content of hyaluronic acid (Hyal-Joint®) on pain relief and quality of life in subjects with knee osteoarthritis: a pilot randomized double-blind placebo-controlled trial. *Nutr J* 2008;7:3.

3. Vázquez JA, Montemayor MI, Fraguas J, et al. Hyaluronic acid production by *Streptococcus zooepidemicus* in marine by-products media from mussel processing wastewaters and tuna peptone viscera. *Microb Cell Fact* 2010;9:46.

4. Cooper C, Brown K, Meletis C, et al. Inflammation and hyaluronic acid. *Altern Compl Ther* 2008;14(2):78–84.

5. Alejandro A, Stamenkovic I, Meinick M, et al. CD44 is the principal cell surface receptor for hyaluronate. *Cell* 1990;61:1303–13.

6. Brown MB, Jones SA. Hyaluronic acid: a unique topical vehicle for the localized delivery of drugs to the skin. *J Eur Acad Dermatol Venereol* 2005;19(3):308–18.

7. Weindl G, Schaller M, Schäfer-Korting M, et al. Hyaluronic acid in the treatment and prevention of skin diseases: molecular biological, pharmaceutical and clinical aspects. *Skin Pharmacol Physiol* 2004;17(5):207–13.

8. Olczyk P, Komosińska-Vassev K, Winsz-Szczotka K, et al. [Hyaluronan: structure, metabolism, functions, and role in wound healing]. *Postepy Hig Med Dosw (Online)*. 2008;62:651–9 [in Polish].

(*PIPER METHYSTICUM*)

Background

Kava is used as an herbal anxiolytic (to relieve anxiety).[1] Clinical trials have shown that the roots and rhizome of kava are safe and effective alternatives to traditional benzodiazepines (diazepam, etc.).[2] Kava may also be helpful for urogenital problems such as interstitial or bacterial cystitis (inflammation of the urinary bladder), prostatitis (inflammation of the prostate gland), muscular relaxation, and the relief of menopausal symptoms.[2,3] These effects are thought to be attributable to anti-inflammatory and analgesic effects of kava on the urogenital tract.[4,5]

The active ingredients in kava are called kavalactones.[6] Although the exact mechanism(s) for kava's activities remains unknown, kavalactones may somehow modify receptor domains rather than interact specifically with receptor binding sites. Other studies suggest that kavalactones act primarily on the limbic system (the part of the brain associated with emotions and drive),[7] and kava may inhibit cytochrome P450 enzymes (which are involved in drug metabolism).[6] Kava may also exert antiseizure effects.[4]

Indications

Suggested Uses in Humans
- Helps control anxiety, insomnia, restlessness
- Controls seizures
- Minimizes urogenital tract inflammation
- Helps patient with muscular pain

Suggested Uses in Dogs and Cats
- Helps control anxiety
- Improves idiopathic cystitis

Recommended Doses

In humans, 45–70 mg of kavalactones q 8 hr is prescribed for use as an anxiolytic or 180–210 mg of kavalactones 1 hr before retiring.[7] In dogs and cats, a 1:2 or 1:3 tincture can be administered at a dose of 0.5–1.5 mL/10 kg/day (divided into three doses).[1] In the author's experience, the dried herb can be administered at 25–75 mg/kg/day (divided into three doses). Alternatively, the following general dosing guidelines can be used in pets: one 100 mg capsule/9 kg dog or 4.5 kg cat q 8–12 hr, 1.25–2.5 mL (¼–½ teaspoon) of powder/11.3 kg dog or 4.5 kg cat q 8–12 hr, or 5–10 drops of a tincture/11.3 kg dog or 4.5 kg cat q 8–12 hr.

Side Effects

Kava is a very safe herb when used as directed. Because of its inhibition of cytochrome P450 enzymes and the potential for hepatotoxicity (especially when combined with other drugs that are known or suspected hepatotoxins), caution is warranted when combining kava with medications or herbs that depend upon cytochrome P450 enzymes for metabolism and/or that exhibit hepatotoxicity as a side effect.[3] Kava dermatopathy syndrome has been described in people (i.e., scale-like lesions on the palms of the hands, soles of the feet, and back).[1] People consuming alcohol should avoid kava usage.[6] There have been reports of severe hepatotoxicity in a few cases of people taking kava. Careful examination of these reports reveals that many of these patients had underlying liver problems, were using hepatotoxic medications, or were drinking alcohol.[3] Additionally, there may have been differences among products containing kava (varying doses or different parts of the kava plant used) or contamination/adulteration of the kava products with hepatotoxic herbs.[6]

Contraindications

Kava should be avoided in patients taking medications, herbs, or other products with known hepatotoxic side effects (e.g., alcohol).

Interactions

Part of the mechanism for kava's efficacy may be weak binding to γ-aminobutyric acid (GABA) and benzodiazepine receptors as well as mixed effects on central dopaminergic pathways. It is therefore prudent to avoid combining kava with benzodiazepines and dopamine agonists or antagonists.[6] Kava may potentiate anticonvulsant medications and increase adverse effects.[6] Large doses of kava may exert a digitalis-like effect (stimulates the heart muscle) and should be avoided in patients taking digitalis glycosides.[5] Avoid kava in patients prescribed proton pump inhibitors (e.g., omeprazole), as coadministration of these medications has been associated with acute hepatitis and liver failure.[6] Theoretically, kava may interact with vitamin K antagonist anticoagulants (such as warfarin), although this has not been proven clinically.[6] As with other herbs that depress the central nervous system, it would be prudent to conclude that kava should be withdrawn approximately 10 days before anesthesia.

References

1. Wynn S, Marsden S. *Manual of natural veterinary medicine: science and tradition*. St. Louis (MO): Mosby; 2003:51–2.

2. Broadfoot PJ, Palmquist RE, Jonston K, et al. *Integrating complementary medicine into veterinary practice*. Goldstein R, ed. Blackwell; 2008:648–9, 687, 697. Available at: www.mediafire.com/?2s13ctmvv7tyb2k. Accessed January 15, 2012.

3. Wynn SG, Fougère B. *Veterinary herbal medicine*. St. Louis (MO): Mosby Elsevier; 2007:377:586–8.

4. Mills S, Bone K. *Principles and practice of phytotherapy: modern herbal medicine*. St. Louis (MO): Churchill Livingstone; 2000:456–63.

5. Fetrow CW, Avila J. *Professional's handbook of complementary and alternative medicines*. 3rd ed. Lippincott Williams & Wilkins; 2004:472.

6. Stargrove M, Treasure J, McKee D. *Herb, nutrient, and drug interactions: clinical implications and therapeutic strategies*. St. Louis (MO): Mosby Elsevier; 2008:106–12.

7. Pizzorno J, Murray M. *Textbook of natural medicine*. 3rd ed. St. Louis (MO): Churchill Livingstone; 2005:1168–72.

Background
Lysine is an essential amino acid (it is not synthesized in the body) that is obtained through the diet by eating meat, poultry, fish, wheat germ, soy, and dairy products.[1] Lysine competes with the amino acid arginine, which is required by viruses for viral replication (particularly herpesviruses).[2] Thus, supplementing with lysine reduces viral replication by competing with arginine (to be absorbed into cells), and can be used in patients infected with feline herpesvirus 1.[3,4] In humans lysine has been used for heartburn, diverticulitis, hypertension, infertility, and as a wound healing aid.[1]

Indications
Suggested Uses in Humans
- Inhibits viral replication in patients with herpes simplex infection
- Improves heartburn and diverticulitis
- Controls hypertension
- Improves infertility
- Aids wound healing

Suggested Uses in Dogs and Cats
- Inhibits viral replication in patients infected with feline herpesvirus 1

Recommended Doses
In humans, 1–6 g/day is recommended for herpes simplex infections.[1] The recommended dose for cats is 250–500 mg *q* 12–24 hr.[4] A similar dose has been recommended in dogs. Regular supplementation with lysine may decrease recurrences of herpesvirus in cats.

Side Effects
High doses may increase the risk for gallstone development and elevate cholesterol levels.[1]

Contraindications

None reported.

Interactions

Lysine and arginine competitively inhibit each other and compete for absorption into cells. Lysine supplementation should be avoided in patients that require additional arginine and vice versa.[2]

References

1. Fetrow CW, Avila J. *Professional's handbook of complementary & alternative medicines*. 3rd ed. Philadelphia (PA): Lippincott Williams & Wilkins; 2004: 524–5.

2. Stargrove M, Treasure J, McKee D. *Herb, nutrient, and drug interactions: clinical implications and therapeutic strategies*. St. Louis (MO): Mosby Elsevier; 2008:659.

3. Broadfoot PJ, Palmquist RE, Jonston K, et al. *Integrating complementary medicine into veterinary practice*. Goldstein R, ed. Blackwell; 2008:612–28. Available at: www.mediafire.com/?2s13ctmvv7tyb2k. Accessed January 15, 2012.

4. Wynn SG, Marsden S. *Manual of natural veterinary medicine: science and tradition*. St. Louis (MO): Mosby; 2003:504, 512, 540.

MEDICINAL MUSHROOMS

(BETA GLUCANS)

Background

There are a number of different mushroom species that have been shown to exhibit various immunostimulating properties. Although it is beyond the scope of this book to examine each of these, some of the species most likely to be used as nutritional supplements are maitake (*Grifola frondosa*), coriolus (*Coriolus versicolor*), reishi (*Ganoderma lucidum)*, agaricus (*Agaricus blazei*), shiitake (*Lentinula edodes*), and cordyceps (*Cordyceps sinensis).* Medicinal mushrooms are useful for general immune support in a variety of medical conditions but are most commonly recommended for patients with cancer. Doctors interested in using these types of supplements can prescribe either medicinal mushrooms or purified beta glucans, the active ingredients in medicinal mushrooms.[1] Beta glucans are polysaccharides (long chains of sugar molecules) and are the major structural components of cell walls of various fungi, including yeast and mushrooms.[1]

As with many supplements, determining the "right dose" is difficult. The chosen dose should result in maximal TNF-α release. However, high concentrations may cause an apparent suppression of TNF-α activity.

Indications

Suggested Uses in Humans

- Supports the immune system
- Helps patients with cancer
- Improves diabetes
- Helps patients with hepatitis and liver diseases
- Controls cystitis
- Acts as a diuretic

Suggested Uses in Dogs and Cats

- Supports the immune system
- Helps patients with cancer

Recommended Doses

Anecdotal doses in people range from 200 mg to 750 mg/day. In dogs and cats, 20–200 mg/0.45 kg/day (divided) is recommended.[2]

Side Effects

Medicinal mushrooms (beta glucan) consumption is considered safe (maitake mushrooms are used in cooking).[2] Because of the possibility of slightly lowering blood glucose levels, there is theoretical concern about the use of beta glucans in diabetic patients taking insulin or oral hypoglycemic medications. These patients should be carefully monitored when coadministered medicinal mushrooms/beta glucan supplements (even though there are no reports of problems in the literature).

Contraindications

None reported. Use should be avoided in patients who are allergic to mushrooms.

Interactions

None reported.

References

1. Pizzorno J, Murray M. *Textbook of natural medicine*. 3rd ed. St. Louis (MO): Churchill Livingstone; 2005:562–3.

2. Wynn SG, Marsden S. *Manual of natural veterinary medicine: science and tradition*. St. Louis (MO): Mosby; 2003:400.

(N-ACETYL-5-METHOXYTRYPTAMINE)

Background

Melatonin is a hormone produced in the brain by the pineal gland via conversion of tryptophan into serotonin and then melatonin.[1] Melatonin is often referred to as the "biological timekeeper" of hormone secretions as it regulates a number of hormones that, in turn, regulate other hormones.[1]

Melatonin production by the pineal gland rises slowly at night and falls during the day in response to increasing dark and light cycles.[1] In addition to the pineal gland, lymphocytes (a type of white blood cell) synthesize and release large amounts of melatonin, inducing restful sleep and acting as an antioxidant.[2] In fact, melatonin is reportedly a potent free radical scavenger that reduces skin damage caused by ultraviolet radiation (when applied topically). Melatonin acts as an antiestrogen hormone, opposes degenerative side effects caused by elevated levels of corticosteroids,[3] and is used in the management of hormone-induced neoplasms.[4] At high doses, melatonin can be used for reducing side effects of as well as enhancing the cytotoxicity of chemotherapy and radiation therapy by promoting apoptosis (programmed cell death of cancer cells) and the release of immunomodulating cytokines (inflammatory mediators).[1,2] Melatonin is involved in regulating the immune system, and increases the beneficial effects of interleukin-2 (IL-2).[1,2] It is also noteworthy that melatonin levels are decreased in pets with Cushing's disease (hyperadrenocorticism).[3]

Melatonin supplements are often either prepared from bovine pineal glands or synthesized from 5-methoxyindole.[5]

Indications

Suggested Uses in Humans
- Induces restful sleep and improves symptoms associated with jet lag
- Acts as a potent antioxidant
- Kills cancer cells

Suggested Uses in Dogs and Cats
- Induces restful sleep

- Acts as a potent antioxidant
- Benefits patients with Cushing's disease
- Kills cancer cells
- Improves various alopecias (e.g., alopecia X, seasonal flank alopecia, boxer alopecia, which are hormone-related disorders)

Recommended Doses

In humans, the typical therapeutic dose is 3 mg/day (range, 0.5–6.0 mg/day). In cancer patients, doses of up to 40 mg/day are used.[1] In dogs and cats, the suggested dose is 1 mg/10 kg body weight/ day to a maximum of 5 mg/animal/day.[3] Alternate doses are 1–5 mg/animal before bed, 3–12 mg q 8–24 hr for alopecia (alopecia X, seasonal flank alopecia, boxer alopecia, which are hormone-related disorders), and 0.2 mg/0.4 kg/day in cancer patients.[6]

Side Effects

Melatonin is generally considered safe when used at the recommended doses. Because it regulates hormones, extended use may interfere with the actions of other hormones. Regular monitoring is advised if melatonin is used for extended periods of time.[1] As expected, excessive drowsiness can occur in patients treated with melatonin, particularly at higher doses.[1] Melatonin may decrease fertility and is not recommended during pregnancy or lactation because of its effects on other hormones and its ability to cross the placenta.[1] Rarely, increased seizure activity in children suffering from neurological disorders after administration of melatonin has been reported.[1]

Contraindications

In humans, contraindications include pregnancy, nursing, depression, patients with nocturnal asthma, adolescents, patients using corticosteroids for anti-inflammatory or immunosuppressive effects (see below), fibromyalgia, and diabetes. Experimental animal research suggests that melatonin may be contraindicated for patients with autoimmune diseases.[1] In a small percentage of people taking melatonin at night to induce restful sleep, the opposite effect is seen and insomnia occurs. Using a lower dose or administering melatonin in the morning may be helpful.[1] If used as a sleep aid, use the lowest effective dose possible, especially for those patients for whom higher doses would be contraindicated.[1]

Interactions

Melatonin may be depleted in patients treated with benzodiazepines; however, melatonin may act synergistically with benzodiazepines (because of a similar mechanism of action) and may permit a dose reduction of the benzodiazepine.[1] Beta-adrenergic antagonists (e.g., propranolol) may suppress melatonin synthesis, especially with chronic use of beta-blockers. Melatonin administration may be beneficial to patients taking beta-blockers, especially those with disturbances in sleep-wake cycles.[1] Administration of corticosteroids may suppress melatonin synthesis, but administering melatonin may counter the side effects of corticosteroids, such as alterations in sleep-wake cycles. Patients taking corticosteroids for immunosuppressive effects should be monitored closely for adverse reactions (e.g., decreased efficacy of corticosteroid therapy) when melatonin is coadministered.[1]

Selective serotonin reuptake inhibitors (SSRIs) such as fluoxetine (prescribed in dogs for separation anxiety, for example) may decrease melatonin levels. Currently there is no recommendation about whether melatonin administration during fluoxetine therapy is recommended or contraindicated.[1] Nonsteroidal anti-inflammatory drug (NSAID, e.g., aspirin) administration may inhibit melatonin synthesis. Therefore, administering melatonin may counter the side effects associated with NSAID administration, including alterations in sleep-wake cycles.[1] Melatonin may also enhance the efficacy and reduce side effects seen with tamoxifen (an antagonist to the estrogen receptor in breast tissue) therapy.[1] Calcium channel blockers (such as verapamil) may result in increased urinary excretion of melatonin, which may disturb sleep-wake cycles. Administering melatonin during calcium channel blocker therapy may be indicated.[1] Because of the possibility of melatonin interfering with the activity of antidepressant medications, its use should probably be avoided in patients taking these medications, or patients should be closely monitored if melatonin is used with antidepressant or antianxiety medications.[1] In laboratory rats, coadministration of melatonin and cyclosporine A may reduce the nephrotoxic effects of the cyclosporine.[1] Finally, caution (or avoidance) with melatonin is indicated in patients taking antihypertensives, as combining the two compounds may result in uncontrolled blood pressure.[1]

References

1. Stargrove M, Treasure J, McKee D. *Herb, nutrient, and drug interactions: clinical implications and therapeutic strategies.* St. Louis (MO): Mosby Elsevier; 2008:769–82.

2. Wynn SG, Marsden S. *Manual of natural veterinary medicine: science and tradition.* St. Louis (MO): Mosby; 2003:399.

3. Broadfoot PJ, Palmquist RE, Jonston K, et al. *Integrating complementary medicine into veterinary practice.* Goldstein R, ed. Blackwell; 2008:42, 513, 515, 787. Available at: www.mediafire.com/?2s13ctmvv7tyb2k. Accessed January 15, 2012.

4. Pizzorno J, Murray M, Joiner-Bey H. *The clinician's handbook of natural medicine.* 2nd ed. St. Louis (MO): Churchill Livingstone; 2008:45, 130, 134.

5. Fetrow CW, Avila J. *Professional's handbook of complementary and alternative Medicines.* 3rd ed. Philadelphia (PA): Lippincott Williams & Wilkins; 2004:515–7.

6. Scott D, Miller W, Griffin C. *Muller and Kirk's small animal dermatology.* 6th ed. Philadelphia (PA): WB Saunders Company; 2001.

METHYLSULFONYLMETHANE

Background

MSM is a natural anti-inflammatory and analgesic supplement that is a metabolite of dimethylsulfoxide (DMSO), which is often recommended for patients with musculoskeletal disorders such as osteoarthritis.[1] MSM also supplies sulfur to the body.[2] Studies in people showed improved joint flexibility, reduced stiffness and swelling, and reduced pain following administration with MSM.[3,4] Animals with rheumatoid arthritis that were given MSM showed no cartilage degeneration. MSM may have other benefits in dogs and cats; however, more research is needed.

Indications

Suggested Uses in Humans
- Improves arthritis
- Supports the musculoskeletal system in the elderly

Suggested Uses in Dogs and Cats
- Improves arthritis
- Supports the musculoskeletal system in the elderly

Recommended Doses

Anecdotal doses in people range from 100 mg 1–3 times/day to 1,000–4,000 mg *q* 12–24 hr. In dogs and cats, one suggested dose of 100–1,000 mg/animal *q* 12–24 hr is recommended.[5] The author has seen some supplements recommending 500–1,000 mg/22.7 kg *q* 12–24 hr.

Side Effects

MSM is considered very safe.[6]

Contraindications

None reported.

Interactions

MSM is often administered in conjunction with glucosamine. There is published evidence supporting the hypothesis that the combination of the two ingredients resulted in a more rapid onset of analgesia (pain relief) and anti-inflammatory effects in patients with osteoarthritis than did either agent alone.[6]

References

1. Fetrow CW, Avila J. *Professional's handbook of complementary and alternative medicines*. 3rd ed. Philadelphia (PA); Lippincott Williams & Wilkins; 2004:557.

2. Kim LS, Axelrod LJ, Howard P, et al. Efficacy of methylsulfonylmethane (MSM) in osteoarthritis pain of the knee: a pilot clinical trial. *Osteoarthritis Cartilage* 2006; 14(3):286–94.

3. Usha PR, Naidu MU. Randomised, double-blind, parallel, placebo-controlled study of oral glucosamine, methylsulfonylmethane, and their combination in osteoarthritis. *Clin Drug Investig* 2004;24(6):353–63.

4. Wynn SG, Marsden S. *Manual of natural veterinary medicine: science and tradition*. St. Louis (MO): Mosby; 2003:341–7.

5. Hixson O. Acute intragastric toxicity (LD-50). Dimethyl sulfone (methylsulfonylmethane, MSM). Laboratory of Vitamin Technology, Inc., Chicago, Illinois, August 21, 1958.

6. Stargrove M, Treasure J, McKee D. *Herb, nutrient, and drug interactions: clinical implications and therapeutic strategies*. St. Louis (MO): Mosby Elsevier; 2008:762.

PHOSPHATIDYLSERINE

Background

Phosphatidylserine is a phospholipid (a long chain of hydrogen and carbon that has a phosphate group on one end) that is an important component of cell membranes where energy is produced for cellular metabolism.[1,2] Phosphatidylserine is particularly important for brain-related functions. It is abundant in tissues of the nervous system and facilitates the initiation of an electrical stimulus during nerve transmission, integrates electrical circuits across the brain, and initiates cell-to-cell nerve stimuli transmission via synapses (the junction between nerves).[2] Phosphatidylserine protects nerve circuits against age-related atrophy.[2]

Given the described mechanisms of action, reports indicate that phosphatidylserine is clinically effective in senile dementia and positively affects anxiety and motivation.[1,3]

Indications

Suggested Uses in Humans
- Improves signs of Alzheimer's disease and dementia

Suggested Uses in Dogs and Cats
- Ameliorates various cognitive disorders

Recommended Doses

The recommended dose in humans is 100 mg *q* 8 hr with food.[3] The recommended dose in dogs and cats is 100–500 mg/day (divided)[4] or 2 mg/kg *q* 12 hr with food.[1]

Side Effects

Phosphatidylserine is considered very safe. Minor side effects such as those seen with phosphatidylcholine supplementation (e.g., gastrointestinal discomfort) may occur rarely.[2] Theoretically, as occurs with choline supplementation in animals, supplementation with phosphatidylserine has the potential to produce excitability/nervousness. Lowering the dose in dogs and cats exhibiting this side effect is indicated. Nonetheless, phosphatidylserine supplementation was well tolerated by dogs administered up to 70 g/day for 1 year.[2]

Contraindications
None reported.

Interactions
None reported.

References

1. Broadfoot PJ, Palmquist RE, Jonston K, et al. *Integrating complementary medicine into veterinary practice.* Goldstein R, ed. Blackwell; 2008:180, 301, 304, 500, 537, 550, 553. Available at: www.mediafire.com/?2s13ctmvv7tyb2k. Accessed January 15, 2012.

2. Pizzorno J, Murray M. *Textbook of natural medicine.* 3rd ed. St. Louis (MO): Churchill Livingstone; 2005:1163–4, 1466–9.

3. Pizzorno J, Murray M, Joiner-Bey H. *The clinician's handbook of natural medicine.* 2nd ed. St. Louis (MO): Churchill Livingstone; 2008:44–7, 599, 604.

4. Wynn SG, Marsden S. *Manual of natural veterinary medicine: science and tradition.* St. Louis (MO): Mosby; 2003:57.

Background

Prebiotics are functional foods (i.e., foods that serve a function, in this case, serving as a nutritive source for probiotics) that contain nondigestible ingredients that benefit the patient by encouraging the growth/activity of one or more symbiotic (beneficial, non-disease-causing) micro-organisms that reside in the gastrointestinal tract. Prebiotics serve as food for the commensal (symbiotic) gastrointestinal bacteria, yeasts, and other micro-organisms.[1] The most common types of prebiotics are long-chain sugar polymers such as fructooligosaccharides (FOSes), which are usually supplied in supplemental form, but are also found in various foods such as asparagus, Globe and Jerusalem artichokes, leeks, onions, and chicory.[2] Other prebiotics are inulin (another long-chain of saccharides); sugar alcohols such as lactitol, maltitol, and xylitol; and galactose oligosaccharides (GOSes).[1]

In addition to serving as a food source for probiotics (the "good" or symbiotic bacteria/commensals in the gastrointestinal tract), supplementation with prebiotics in people inhibits the growth of pathogens (disease-causing organisms), modulates immune development by favoring T-helper cell 1 (TH1) and inhibiting T-helper cell 2 (TH2), and may play a role in reducing or preventing allergies (e.g., eczema, atopic dermatitis), especially when administered to infants.[1]

Indications

Suggested Uses in Humans
- Supports the immune system
- Contributes to the health of the gastrointestinal tract
- Feeds probiotics and commensal gastrointestinal micro-organisms

Suggested Uses in Dogs and Cats
- Supports the immune system
- Contributes to the health of the gastrointestinal tract
- Feeds probiotics and commensal gastrointestinal micro-organisms

Recommended Doses

In humans, a typical dose of FOS is 5–20 g/day (usually q 8–12 hr with meals). Specific doses in dogs and cats do not appear to be published as yet.

Side Effects

Prebiotics are extremely safe. To date, no safety issues have been published. At higher doses, they can cause bloating, flatulence, and gastrointestinal discomfort in people. Mild side effects are common, but are less common at lower doses and decrease over time.[2]

Contraindications

None reported.

Interactions

Some experts trained in nutritional therapeutics recommend "fertilizing" the gastrointestinal tract with prebiotics before starting probiotics. This is thought to maximize the effectiveness of probiotic therapy.[3]

References

1. Broadfoot PJ, Palmquist RE, Jonston K, et al. *Integrating complementary medicine into veterinary practice.* Goldstein R, ed. Blackwell; 2008:372. Available at: www.mediafire.com/?2s13ctmvv7tyb2k. Accessed January 15, 2012.

2. Pizzorno J, Murray M. *Textbook of natural medicine.* 3rd ed. St. Louis (MO): Churchill Livingstone; 2005:1185–7, 1191.

3. Stargrove M, Treasure J, McKee D. *Herb, nutrient, and drug interactions: clinical implications and therapeutic strategies.* St. Louis (MO): Mosby Elsevier; 2008:815, 822–3.

Background

Probiotics are living nonpathogenic bacteria and yeasts. Typical probiotic bacteria include various species of *Bifidobacterium* (e.g., *B. bifidus*), *Lactobacillus* (e.g., *L. acidophilus*), *Streptococcus* (e.g., *S. thermophilus*), and *Enterococcus* (e.g., *E. faecium*). Probiotic yeasts include *Saccharomyces* (e.g., *S. bulgaricus*).[1] Probiotics can also be found in live-culture foods such as yogurt and kefir.[1] The function of probiotics is to improve the "balance" of the intestinal microflora by favoring the growth of nonpathogenic (non-disease-causing) organisms in the gastrointestinal tract.[2] Positive benefits associated with probiotics include increased endogenous synthesis of vitamins (e.g., B vitamins and vitamin K); enhanced synthesis of short-chain fatty acids and amino acids; reduced intestinal permeability; reduction in antimicrobial-induced diarrhea (especially from treating *Clostridium difficile* infections); enhanced immune function (possibly by preventing or controlling asthma, allergies, systemic infections, and autoimmune disorders); reduced serum cholesterol; and improvement in various gastrointestinal disorders (e.g., diarrhea, irritable bowel syndrome, inflammatory bowel syndrome, "leaky gut," *Helicobacter pylori* infection, gastrointestinal parasitism, etc).[1,2] Other suggested mechanism of action include increased secretory immunoglobulin A (IgA), promoting cytokine (inflammatory mediator) synthesis to improve the gastrointestinal environment, restoring normal intestinal flora (population of micro-organisms in the gastrointestinal tract), and producing metabolites such as hydroxide that are toxic to pathogenic bacteria. Finally, probiotics purportedly neutralize dietary carcinogens.[1]

Probiotics can be administered either with or following therapy with various medications, including antibiotics, antifungals, corticosteroids, nonsteroidal anti-inflammatory drugs (NSAIDs, e.g., aspirin), and cancer chemotherapeutic agents.[1] Improperly stored or outdated probiotic products may not be efficacious because of breakdown of the micro-organism(s).[3] In the author's experience, such products may cause minor gastrointestinal distress and nausea. In order for a probiotic to be efficacious, living micro-organisms must be present in the products, and viable micro-organisms must survive passage through the acidic environment of the stomach and adhere to the intestinal epithelium in order to exert a beneficial effect.[4]

There is some debate about whether pets need different strains of micro-organisms in their probiotics supplement than humans. Unfortunately, more research is needed before this question can be answered. At this time, it appears that the use of any probiotic product may help both people and pets. For example, *Lactobacilli* spp., *Enterococci* spp., and *Bifidobacteria* spp. are all part of the normal gastrointestinal microflora of healthy dogs and cats (like humans), and probiotic supplements containing these species may be effective in those species.[5] Laboratory analysis of various probiotic products, including pet foods that claim to contain probiotics, often fail to find viable micro-organisms in the products. Specifically, one study examined 19 commercial pet foods claiming to contain probiotics. Not one of the products contained all of the listed organisms, and no relevant growth of bacteria on culture media was present in 5 out of 19 (26%) products. Average bacterial growth ranged from 0 to 1.8×10^5 colon-forming units/g (which is at the low end of the recommended dose of probiotics for people and pets). That study concluded that the probiotic content of the diets was not accurately represented by the label descriptions. Additionally, the labels of five pet foods had misspellings of the names of the micro-organisms contained in the food, raising concerns about the quality of the products.[6]

The company ConsumerLab.com recently reported the results of their analysis of both human and pet probiotic supplements.[7] Only 2 out of 13 human probiotic products accurately listed the number of viable micro-organisms on their labels. For pet probiotic products, very large differences were noted in the number of micro-organisms in the supplements compared with the suggested daily doses on the labels. Results of those studies do not necessarily suggest that the products were inaccurately or fraudulently labeled at the time of manufacturing, although that is certainly possible. A large percentage of organisms in a probiotic supplement may die before a product is even purchased. Products should be stored in sealed containers and away from heat, light, and humidity. In addition, if a label indicates that a product should be refrigerated prior to opening, it should be sold in a refrigerated condition and kept that way. Probiotic products should be purchased from reputable manufacturers and stored according to manufacturer recommendations.[3]

Indications

Suggested Uses in Humans

- Supports gastrointestinal health (e.g., patients with *H. pylori* infection) and protects against diarrhea, including antibiotic-induced diarrhea, traveler's diarrhea, chemotherapy-induced diarrhea, irritable bowel syndrome, inflammatory bowel disease, and Crohn's disease
- Protects against "leaky gut" syndrome
- Improves *Candida* infections (especially vaginal)
- Helps patients with allergies (e.g., eczema, atopic dermatitis, food allergies)

Suggested Uses in Dogs and Cats

- Supports gastrointestinal health (e.g., patients with *H. pylori* infection) and protects against diarrhea, including antibiotic-induced diarrhea, traveler's diarrhea, chemotherapy-induced diarrhea, irritable bowel syndrome, inflammatory bowel disease, and Crohn's disease
- Protects against "leaky gut" syndrome
- Helps patients with allergies (e.g., eczema, atopic dermatitis, food allergies)

Recommended Doses

Successful results in people have been attained using between 10^7 and 10^{11} viable bacteria/day.[4] Dose requirements for probiotic organisms have not been evaluated adequately in dogs and cats and they may vary among different probiotic strains. Conventionally, a minimum of 10^6 viable micro-organisms (colony-forming units) is recommended. According to one source, 500 million colony-forming units/11.4 kg is appropriate.[8]

Side Effects

Probiotics are among the safest supplements currently available for people and pets. In humans, mild flu-like symptoms, flatulence, bloating, loose stools, and nausea can occur. If side effects do occur, they usually develop within the first 1–2 weeks of administration. Clinical signs can be alleviated by reducing the dose of probiotics or temporarily stopping the supplement.[1]

Contraindications

If probiotics are used in people and pets with immunosuppressive conditions, there is a slight (theoretical) possibility of infection with any of the micro-organisms contained in the probiotic supplement.[1]

Interactions

Various herbs (ginseng, etc.) may require the action of intestinal micro-organisms to become biologically active. Probiotic administration may therefore enhance the activity of these herbs (which otherwise might not be activated to their active forms in the absence of normal gastrointestinal microflora).[1] Echinacea may stimulate the growth of certain pathogenic *Bacteroides* organisms and probiotic administration may counteract this effect.[1]

In vitro, *L. acidophilus* may accelerate the metabolism of sulfasalazine, although this has not been noted *in vivo*.[1]

Some experts trained in nutritional therapeutics recommend "fertilizing" the gastrointestinal tract with prebiotics before starting the probiotics. This is thought to maximize the effectiveness of probiotic therapy.[1]

References

1. Stargrove M, Treasure J, McKee D. *Herb, nutrient, and drug interactions: clinical implications and therapeutic strategies.* St. Louis (MO): Mosby Elsevier; 2008:815–23.

2. Wynn SG, Marsden S. *Manual of natural veterinary medicine: science and tradition.* St. Louis (MO): Mosby; 2003:163, 184, 193–4, 271.

3. Fetrow CW, Avila J. *Professional's handbook of complementary and alternative medicines.* 3rd ed. Philadelphia (PA): Lippincott Williams & Wilkins; 2004:15.

4. Pizzorno J, Murray M. *Textbook of natural medicine.* 3rd ed. St. Louis (MO): Churchill Livingstone; 2005:1195–1209.

5. Hand M, Thatcher C, Remillard R, et al. *Small animal clinical nutrition.* 5th ed. Topeka (KS): Mark Morris Institute; 2010:761.

6. Weese JS, Arroyo L. Bacteriological evaluation of dog and cat diets that claim to contain probiotics. *Can Vet J* 2003:44(3):212–5. Available at: http://www.ncbi.nlm.nih.gov/pmc/articles/PMC340078/pdf/20030300s00016p212.pdf. Accessed February 20, 2012.

7. ConsumerLab.com. Product review: probiotics for adults, children and pets. Available at: https://www.consumerlab.com/reviews/Probiotic_Supplements_Lactobacillus_acidophilus_Bifidobacterium/probiotics/. Accessed February 21, 2012.

8. Broadfoot PJ, Palmquist RE, Jonston K, et al. *Integrating complementary medicine into veterinary practice.* Goldstein R, ed. Blackwell; 2008:240, 298. Available at: www.mediafire.com/?2s13ctmvv7tyb2k. Accessed January 15, 2012.

S-ADENOSYLMETHIONINE

Background

SAMe is formed in the body (mainly in the liver) from the amino acid methionine and adenosine triphosphate (ATP, the body's storage form of energy). SAMe is therefore an essential nutrient, not supplied in the diet.[1] SAMe functions as a methyl donor (one carbon and three hydrogen molecules) to assist in the formation of a variety of compounds such as neurotransmitters, proteins, membrane phospholipids, nucleic acids, and choline.[1,2] After donating a methyl group, SAMe is converted to S-adenosylhomocysteine (SAH), which, in turn, donates sulfur to form amino acids (e.g., taurine, glutathione, cysteine), donates adenosine, and is then rapidly metabolized to homocysteine.[1]

A number of trials have examined the benefits of SAMe. These studies suggest that SAMe increases levels of serotonin and dopamine metabolites. Thus, SAMe supplementation in people with depression purportedly increases the neurotransmitters serotonin and dopamine, improves neuron membrane fluidity, improves binding of neurotransmitters to receptors, and reduces signs of depression like the tricyclic antidepressants (TCAs).[2] In arthritic patients, SAMe is utilized in cartilage synthesis, shows mild analgesic and anti-inflammatory effects, and reduces medical symptoms as well as or greater than nonsteroidal anti-inflammatory drugs (NSAIDs).[2] SAMe has a beneficial effect on the liver and may enhance the elimination of certain drugs (e.g., acetaminophen).[3] SAMe showed an effectiveness in preventing gastric mucosal injury similar to that of the pharmaceutical drug misoprostol in rodent studies. This protective effect was thought to be because of increased synthesis of nonprotein sulfhydryl compounds in the gastrointestinal tract.[4] Finally, SAMe has an anti-inflammatory action and improves liver function in less severe cases of cirrhosis (scarring).[5]

SAMe levels decline and are typically low in the elderly. In addition, SAMe levels are often low in patients with osteoarthritis, depression, and various liver disorders.[3] Because of the first pass effect (i.e., it is metabolized first by the gastric and liver enzymes before reaching the target site, resulting in a decreased concentration of the compound in circulation), SAMe is poorly absorbed and has poor bioavailability.[4] The major drawback of SAMe supplementation is its expense.

Indications

Suggested Uses in Humans

- Improves depression
- Improves Alzheimer's
- Helps patients with epilepsy
- Supports patients with arthritis
- Helps patients with multiple sclerosis and spinal cord disease
- Offers liver support and decreases severity of intoxications (e.g., acetaminophen)

Suggested Uses in Dogs and Cats

- Offers liver support and decreases severity of intoxications (e.g., acetaminophen)
- Improves cognitive disorders
- Supports patients with arthritis

Recommended Doses

In humans, 1,200 mg/day (usually 400 mg *q* 6–8 hr) is most often used in clinical trials. In practice, the most common dose is 400 mg/day, likely because of the high cost of the supplement.[1] In dogs and cats, the recommended dose is 10–20 mg/kg/day.[5]

Side Effects

Approximately 20% of people taking SAMe develop side effects. Most side effects are minor and associated with the gastrointestinal tract (e.g., dry mouth, nausea) or skin (rashes).[1] Restlessness has also been observed. People with a history of bipolar/manic disorder(s) should avoid SAMe because of a possible risk of a manic or hypomanic episode.[1] Homocysteine levels may be elevated during SAMe supplementation. Elevated homocysteine levels place individuals at risk for coronary disease and thrombosis.[1] The safety of SAMe administration in infants and children has not been evaluated.[1] Similar concerns may exist for dogs and cats; however, there are currently no reports of serious side effects associated with SAMe supplementation.

Contraindications

In people, contraindications include bipolar disorder, migraine headaches, Parkinson's disease, and in patients with active bleeding. Caution is warranted in people with coronary artery disease, as SAMe is a precursor to homocysteine and elevated homocysteine levels have been implicated in coronary artery disease.[1] No direct contraindications are currently noted in dogs and cats.

Interactions

Caution should be exercised in patients taking monoamine oxidase (MAO) inhibitors, foods with high tyramine content, and certain opioid derivatives such as meperidine and dextromethorphan because of possible interactions. SAMe and tricyclic antidepressants (TCAs) exert similar influences on the central nervous system. Thus, when they are used together, an additive or synergistic effect may be noted, potentially resulting in an excessive pharmacologic response. Caution should be taken if patients taking TCAs are also prescribed SAMe.[1] In people, SAMe may contribute to Parkinsonian-like motor impairments by interfering with the action of L-dopa. Although some patients with Parkinson's disease may benefit from SAMe, others may have their symptoms exacerbated by administration of SAMe.[1] In women, SAMe acts as an "antidote" against hepatobiliary toxicity caused by estrogen administration (i.e., oral contraceptives).[1]

SAMe supplementation may result in a synergistic or additive effect on hepatobiliary function when given with ursodeoxycholic acid (Ursodiol, a drug used to reduce symptoms associated with severe hepatobiliary disease).[1] Patients with active bleeding disorders or taking anticoagulants should use SAMe with caution because of the possibility of increased bleeding.[1] Finally, coadministration of SAMe and selective serotonin reuptake inhibitors (SSRIs, used as antidepressants and antipsychotics) can enhance the effectiveness of treatment for depression. Caution must be used, as some patients may be at a higher risk of serotonin syndrome, a potentially life-threatening condition associated with increased serotonin levels.[1] Extreme caution should be taken when SAMe is combined with MAO inhibitors (e.g., selegiline) because of the theoretical possibility of severe side effects (despite the lack of published evidence that such side effects have occurred).[1] Finally, caution should be used when administering SAMe with

5-hydroxytyptophan (5-HTP) or other supplements or herbs with an antidepressant effect because of the theoretical possibility of an interaction between the supplements.[1]

References

1. Stargrove M, Treasure J, McKee D. *Herb, nutrient, and drug interactions: clinical implications and therapeutic strategies.* St. Louis (MO): Mosby Elsevier; 2008:824–1.

2. Pizzorno J, Murray M, Joiner-Bey H. The clinician's handbook of natural medicine. 2nd ed. St. Louis (MO): Churchill Livingstone; 2008:17, 20, 559–60.

3. Pizzorno J, Murray M. Textbook of natural medicine. 3rd ed. St. Louis (MO): Churchill Livingstone; 2005:1235–8.

4. Fetrow CW, Avila J. *Professional's handbook of complementary and alternative medicines.* 3rd ed. Philadelphia (PA): Lippincott Williams & Wilkins: 2004:730–58.

5. Broadfoot PJ, Palmquist RE, Jonston K, et al. *Integrating complementary medicine into veterinary practice.* Goldstein R, ed. Blackwell; 2008:348, 605, 607. Available at: www.mediafire.com/?2s13ctmvv7tyb2k. Accessed January 15, 2012.

SILYMARIN/MILK THISTLE

(*SILYBUM MARIANUM*)

Background

Milk thistle, occasionally called holy thistle or St. Mary's thistle, contains silymarin—a complex of silibinin (silybin), isosilybin, silidianin, and silychristin. Silibinin is the primary compound; however, other ingredients are also present, such as apigenin, histamine, oleic acid, stearic acid, palmitic acid, and myristic acid.[1,2]

Silymarin inhibits several liver enzymes, including cytochrome P450 (CYP450), CYP3A4-, and CYP2C9- *in vitro*, which are enzymes involved in drug metabolism.[2] Theoretically, because many hepatotoxins require activation by CYP enzymes, any compound that inhibits cytochrome enzymes would reduce or eliminate the toxicity of the hepatotoxins. More research is needed to determine clinical implications. Silymarin may also induce hepatic cytochrome enzymes and therefore increase the clearance of certain drugs (such as metronidazole), resulting in reduced plasma levels and possible decreased drug efficacy.[1] Studies have also shown that silymarin protects the liver from damage by cyclopeptide-containing mushrooms (e.g., *Amanita, Galerina,* and *Lepiota* spp.);[3] however, a clinical response usually requires intravenous administration of silymarin (which is not always clinically feasible).[4] The hepatoregenerative ability of silymarin occurs through stimulation of RNA polymerase A, which may enhance ribosome protein synthesis and cell development.[5] Silymarin also exerts a hepatoprotective effect by altering the outer hepatocyte cell membrane so that toxins cannot enter the cell.[1] Silymarin causes an increase in low-density lipoprotein (LDL, "bad") cholesterol, a decrease in liver cholesterol concentration, and a decreased level of serum cholesterol.[1] Silymarin acts as an antioxidant/free radical scavenger.[6] Thus, administration increases the intracellular concentration of the antioxidants glutathione and superoxide dismutase,[7] and inhibits the formation of leukotrienes (inflammatory mediators) by inhibiting the 5-lipoxygenase (5-LOX) pathway. Supplementation with silymarin is also thought to increases bile flow (choleretic activity).[1] In addition, silymarin modulates P-glycoprotein (a transport protein) and exerts an anticirrhotic effect by inhibiting transformation of hepatocytes into fibroblasts.[6] Silymarin administration is often used to improve/normalize elevated liver enzymes and chelate heavy metals.[7] Silymarin is also considered a chemopreventive agent by inhibiting intestinal beta-glucuronidases, modulating carcinogen metabolizing enzymes, and inhibiting epidermal growth factor receptor and kinases.[1] Silymarin inhibits the growth of certain human cancer lines *in vitro*, and topical application of silymarin reduces tumor formation in laboratory mice.[1] Finally, one recent meta-analysis found that *Silybum marianum* may in fact improve glycemic control in type 2 diabetes, as widely hypothesized.[8]

Commercial supplements are prepared from the seeds (also called the fruit) of *S. marianum*.[3] Extracts are usually standardized to 70% silymarin.[6] It should be noted that the bioavailability of silibinin in milk thistle supplements is extremely low.

Indications
Suggested Uses in Humans
- Supports the liver, decreases liver enzymes, and serves as an antidote for hepatotoxins
- Exerts antineoplastic effects
- Minimizes diabetic complications in people

Suggested Uses in Dogs and Cats
- Supports the liver, decreases liver enzymes, and serves as an antidote for hepatotoxins
- Exerts antineoplastic effects

Recommended Doses
In humans, the recommended dose is 200–800 mg *q* 24 hr or *q* 8–12 hr of the standardized extract. Thus, a 20 g dose of milk thistle standardized to 70% silymarin/silibinin contains 140 mg of silymarin/silibinin.[1] In dogs and cats, administer 10–15 mg/kg/day (divided) of the dry extract (standardized to 70% silymarin) or 1–2 mL/10 kg (divided) of a 1:1 extract.[5] In the author's experience, higher doses can be used to treat intoxications (start with 100–300 mg/11.3–22.7 kg *q* 12 hr).

Side Effects
Milk thistle/silymarin is regarded as a very safe supplement with only very rare side effects, such as a mild laxative effect and uterine stimulation.[7] Allergies are also possible but only rarely reported.[1]

Contraindications

Caution should be used in patients with known hypersensitivity to plants belonging to the *Asteraceae* family.[1]

Interactions

Because of possible inhibition or induction of hepatic cytochrome enzymes, drugs metabolized by cytochrome enzymes may be inhibited or have reduced plasma concentrations and patients should be monitored closely. Silymarin reduces the nephrotoxicity of cisplatin and carboplatin without reducing their effectiveness. This action can possibly increase the effectiveness of these chemotherapeutic agents in certain cancers. In fact, silymarin may actually sensitize certain cancers to treatment with this class of chemotherapeutic agents.[1] Silymarin may reduce adverse effects of anthracyclines, such as doxorubicin, by reducing lipid peroxidation and by stabilizing membranes. Insulin requirements in patients with type 1 diabetes mellitus may be reduced by administration of silymarin. There may also be a protective effect in type 1 and type 2 diabetics.[1] One study in dogs found an increased efficacy of metronidazole when coadministered with silymarin for giardiasis.[1] Finally, one nutritional supplement that contains a combination of silibinin and phosphatidylcholine reportedly increases plasma levels of silibinin.[2]

References

1. Stargrove M, Treasure J, McKee D. *Herb, nutrient, and drug interactions: clinical implications and therapeutic strategies.* St. Louis (MO): Mosby Elsevier; 2008:123–30.

2. Fetrow CW, Avila J. *Professional's handbook of complementary and alternative medicines.* 3rd ed. Philadelphia (PA): Lippincott Williams & Wilkins; 2004:558–62.

3. Wynn SG, Fougère B. *Veterinary herbal medicine.* St. Louis (MO): Mosby Elsevier; 2007:332, 600–2.

4. Schoen A, Wynn SG. *Complementary and alternative veterinary medicine: principles and practice.* St. Louis (MO): Mosby; 1998:323, 351–2.

5. Wynn SG, Marsden S. *Manual of natural veterinary medicine: science and tradition.* St. Louis (MO): Mosby; 2003:317–31.

6. Mills S, Bone K. *Principles and practice of phytotherapy: modern herbal medicine.* St. Louis (MO): Churchill Livingstone: 2000:553–62.

7. Pizzorno J, Murray M. *Textbook of natural medicine*. 3rd ed. St. Louis (MO): Churchill Livingstone; 2005:125–35.

8. Suksomboon N, Poolsup N, Boobkaew S, et al. Meta-analysis of the effect of herbal supplement on glycemic control in type 2 diabetes. J *Ethnopharmacol* 2011;137(3):1328–33.

ST. JOHN'S WORT

(SJW, *HYPERICUM PERFORATUM*)

Background

The flowering tops of St. John's wort (SJW) were traditionally used to relieve anxiety and depression as well as internally and externally for pain relief.[1-3] The herb contains a number of active ingredients, including hypericin, hyperforin, essential oils, and proanthocyanins (secondary plant metabolites).[2]

SJW exhibits several significant pharmacologic interactions that affect drug metabolism, including cytochrome P450 and other cytochrome oxidases that are involved in drug metabolism, transporter proteins, and conjugases and transferases (involved in metabolic reactions). Therefore, this herb directly affects various stages of drug metabolism and detoxification for many drugs.[3] SJW induces P-glycoprotein (a transporter protein) and activates the nuclear receptor called pregnane X receptor (PXR), which induces detoxification of toxic compounds.[3]

In addition to those mentioned above, SJW has several unusual and complex mechanisms of action. As an antidepressant, hyperforin (and likely other constituents) act as an uptake inhibitor for the neurotransmitters serotonin, noradrenaline, dopamine-L-glutamate, and γ-aminobutyric acid (GABA).[1,4]

SJW has been shown to be as effective as traditional (pharmaceutical) antidepressants for patients with mild to moderate depression, usually accompanied by fewer side effects.[2] In addition, hypericin exhibits antiviral activity as well as broad-spectrum antibacterial activity.[4] In HIV/AIDs patients, SJW inhibits protein kinase C and viral production.[5]

Indications

Suggested Uses in Humans

- Functions as an antidepressant
- Helps patients with seasonal affective disorder (SAD)
- Improves insomnia
- Possesses antimicrobial activities (e.g., against HIV)

Suggested Uses in Dogs and Cats

- Functions as an antidepressant

Recommended Doses

Suggested doses in humans are 2–5 g/day of the dried plant, 1–3 mL/day of the tincture or fluid extract, and 900 mg/day (divided, typically 300 mg *q* 8 hr) of a standardized (0.3% hypericin) extract.[3] In dogs and cats, the following general guidelines have been recommended: 25–30 mg/kg/day (divided), 0.5–1.5 mL of 1:2–1:3 tincture/10 kg (divided).[2]

Side Effects

Phototoxicity/photosensitization is a possible adverse effect of SJW in both humans and animals,[1] and is a recognized side effect called hypericism in herbivores that consume SJW. Photosensitization is unlikely to develop in patients prescribed standard doses of SJW.[6] Nonetheless, it may be prudent to limit overexposure to the sun. Caution is warranted when combining SJW with other medications, especially conventional antidepressants (see below).[7] Because of the numerous potential drug interactions with SJW, caution is always advised when using conventional medications and SJW, especially those conventional medications (or herbs) with similar mechanisms of action. It may be prudent to slowly introduce/slowly reduce/taper the dose of any drug or herb that is coadministered with SJW.[3] As mentioned above, SJW works through several unusual and complex mechanisms and acts as an uptake inhibitor for serotonin, noradrenaline, dopamine L-glutamate, and GABA. Interactions with medications or herbs that also inhibit the reuptake of these neurotransmitters is possible.[6]

Contraindications

No specific contraindications exist, but numerous potential safety issues and interactions are described (see "Side Effects" and "Interactions" sections).

Interactions

SJW lowers plasma levels of benzodiazepines (e.g., alprazolam, midazolam, and diazepam) because of cytochrome P4 50 induction. Regular monitoring of blood levels and adjusting doses of benzodiazepines are needed.[3] SJW should be avoided in patients prescribed tricyclic antidepressants (TCAs) and antiretroviral medications because of probable negative interactions.[1] Caution is warranted when SJW is prescribed to patients taking monoamine oxidase (MAO) inhibitors and selective serotonin reuptake inhibitors (SSRIs).[3] SJW may be used safely with general anesthesia; caution is warranted, as SJW may interact with benzodiazepines and anesthetic drugs (especially halogenated anesthetics). Cessation of SJW approximately 10 days prior to anesthesia (to allow complete reversal of enzyme induction) is suggested.[3]

Administration of SJW to patients taking cyclosporine will result in significant reduction in blood levels of cyclosporine. Careful monitoring of circulating levels of cyclosporine is recommended.[1,3] Short-term increases in digoxin levels may occur in patients coadministered SJW. In addition, long-term use of SJW in patients taking digoxin may result in a decline in digoxin levels.[3] SJW may also reduce levels of the chemotherapeutic imatinib, a tyrosine kinase inhibitor, and interfere with the actions of microtubule stabilizing chemotherapy medications (e.g., paclitaxel) because of induction of hepatic cytochrome enzymes.[3] SJW may lower serum levels of omeprazole and other proton pump inhibitors as well as certain statin drugs because of increased metabolism.[3] In contrast, serum levels of tacrolimus (an immunosuppressant drug) may be decreased with SJW because of increased metabolism. Please note that the nephrotoxicity of tacrolimus increases if the tacrolimus dose was increased to compensate for the decreased serum levels during coadministration of SJW. Therefore, the combination of tacrolimus and SJW should be avoided.[3] Serum levels of verapamil and other calcium channel blockers may also decrease when administered with SJW, as well as serum levels of triazole antifungal medications (e.g., itraconazole, fluconazole) because of enzyme induction by SJW.[3] Finally, decreased levels of warfarin or other vitamin K antagonist anticoagulants can be decreased when coadministered with SJW. Careful monitoring of patients using anticoagulants and SJW is necessary.[3]

Please note that the homeopathic dilutions of SJW are useful for nerve pain and trauma. The precautions and potential drug-herb interactions listed above do not apply to homeopathic dilutions.[1]

References

1. Wynn SG, Marsden S. *Manual of natural veterinary medicine: science and tradition.* St. Louis (MO): Mosby; 2003:52, 67, 150, 460, 480.

2. Wynn SG, Fougère B. *Veterinary herbal medicine.* St. Louis (MO): Mosby Elsevier; 2007:1–3, 345, 355, 643–5.

3. Stargrove M, Treasure J, McKee D. *Herb, nutrient, and drug interactions: clinical implications and therapeutic strategies.* St. Louis (MO): Mosby Elsevier; 2008:140–59.

4. Broadfoot PJ, Palmquist RE, Jonston K, et al. *Integrating complementary medicine into veterinary practice.* Goldstein R, ed. Blackwell; 2008:647, 700. Available at: www.mediafire.com/?2s13ctmvv7tyb2k. Accessed January 15, 2012.

5. Pizzorno J, Murray M, Joiner-Bey H. *The clinician's handbook of natural medicine.* 2nd ed. St. Louis (MO): Churchill Livingstone; 2008:320, 333.

6. Mills S, Bone K. *Principles and practice of phytotherapy: modern herbal medicine.* St. Louis (MO): Churchill Livingstone; 2000:542–50.

7. Fetrow CW, Avila J. *Professional's handbook of complementary & alternative medicines.* 3rd ed. Philadelphia (PA): Lippincott Williams & Wilkins; 2004:798–802.

SUPER GREEN FOODS: SPIRULINA/BLUE-GREEN ALGAE

(*SPIRULINA PLATENSIS, S. MAXIMA*)

Background

Spirulina spp. are components of "super foods" that contain amino acids, peptides, proteins, vitamins, minerals, sugars, fatty acids (25–30% γ-linolenic acid [GLA] compared with only 10–15% GLA for evening primrose oil), and nucleic acids.[1] *Spirulina* are blue-green algae with immune-enhancing properties.[1] For example, *Spirulina* enhance natural killer (a type of infection-fighting white blood cell) functions.[1] One compound isolated from *Spirulina* called C-phycocyanin (C-PC, a protein found in certain bacteria and algae that capture light) possesses potent antioxidant, anti-inflammatory, anticancer (via induction of apoptosis), and antiviral properties.[1]

Supplements made with these super foods may vary in their exact compositions as a result of cultivation, harvesting, and processing.[1]

Indications

Suggested Uses in Humans

- Helps patients with cancer
- Reduces radiation/chemotherapy side effects
- Fights infection
- Supports the liver
- Helps patients with either Crohn's disease/ulcerative colitis or constipation
- Improves ulcers
- Alleviates halitosis

Suggested Uses in Dogs and Cats

- Provides general nutritional support
- Supports the immune system
- Fights infection
- Helps patients with cancer

Recommended Doses

Between 200 mg and 500 mg q 8 hr has been recommended in humans.[1] In dogs and cats, super green foods are most commonly used as a general nutritional supplement. Use the dose recommended on the label of the specific product chosen.

Side Effects

Super (green) foods are "generally regarded as safe"; however, some safety concerns exist. First, certain species of *Spirulina* produce toxins that can contaminate nutritional supplements, making them unsafe for consumption.[2] Second, *Spirulina* may contain mercury, which is a toxic heavy metal.[1]

Contraindications

None reported.

Interactions

There are some potential interactions, but none have been clinically proven to date. There is the potential for antagonism with vitamin K antagonist anticoagulants such as warfarin because of the high vitamin K content of green foods. It has also been suggested that green foods may potentially interact with immunosuppressant medications and angiotensin 1 converting enzyme (ACE) inhibitors (which are used to help control blood pressure).

References

1. Fetrow CW, Avila J. *Professional's handbook of complementary and alternative medicines.* 3rd ed. Philadelphia (PA): Lippincott Williams & Wilkins; 2004:787–90.

2. Habib M, Parvin M, Huntington TC, et al. A review on culture, production and use of *Spirulina* as food for humans and feeds for domestic animals and fish. FAO Fisheries and Aquaculture Circular No. 1034. 2008. Available at: ftp://ftp.fao.org/docrep/fao/011/i0424e/i0424e00.pdf. Accessed March 12, 2012.

Background

Taurine is a nonessential sulfur-containing amino acid found naturally in meat, fish, and milk.[1] Taurine synthesis occurs in the liver and the brain from the amino acid cysteine.[2] In fact, taurine is one of the most abundant amino acids in the mammalian brain.[1]

Taurine functions with γ-aminobutyric acid (GABA) and the amino acid glycine as a neuroinhibitory transmitter. It also protects/stabilizes brain cell membranes and exhibits antianxiety and anticonvulsant activity, making it useful for the treatment of seizures.[3]

In addition to the above-described mechanisms of action, taurine acts as a metabolic transmitter, exerts a detoxifying effect, strengthens cardiac contractility, and plays an important role in bile acid metabolism (it is incorporated into bile acids).[3] In cats taurine is the only conjugate for bile acids, whereas the livers of other species are also able to use glycine.[2,4] Taurine is essential in cats' diets. It is also noteworthy that in cats, taurine deficiency was determined to be the primary cause of dilated cardiomyopathy (in 1987). As a result, the Association of American Feed Control Officials (AAFCO) revised taurine requirements in cat food: dry food should have a minimum of 0.1% taurine and wet food should have a minimum of 0.2% taurine.[2] Taurine is helpful in the treatment of retinal degeneration in cats as well as heart disease, cardiac arrhythmias, and congestive heart failure.[4]

Indications

Suggested Uses in Humans

- Helps manage heart disease
- Reduces seizures

Suggested Uses in Dogs and Cats

- Minimizes chances of developing dilated cardiomyopathy
- Protects against retinal degeneration (cats)
- Reduces seizures

Recommended Doses

In humans, the recommended dose is 750 mg q 34 hr for intractable epilepsy.[1] In dogs and cats, a dose range of 50–1,000 mg q 24 hr (or 50–100 mg/kg q 8–24 hr) is recommended. For cocker spaniel cardiomyopathy, a suggested dose is 500 mg q 8 hr.[4]

Side Effects

Taurine is a very safe supplement. Reported side effects in people include diarrhea and constipation.

Contraindications

None reported.

Interactions

Two interactions are worth noting here. First, a beneficial effect of cosupplementing iron-deficient human female patients with iron deficiency anemia with both taurine and slow-release iron was noted.[5] Second, an "amplifying" effect of taurine supplementation on the synthesis of cytochrome P450 enzymes (involved in drug metabolism) and urinary excretion of vitamin C has been reported. This finding suggests that taurine supplementation may have potentially significant clinically effects on drugs or chemicals that are metabolized by those enzymes.[5]

References

1. Pizzorno J, Murray M. *Textbook of Natural Medicine*. 3rd ed. Churchill Livingstone Elsevier; 2005:1654.

2. Hand M, Thatcher C, Remillard R, et al. *Small animal clinical nutrition*. 5th ed. Topeka (KS): Mark Morris Institute; 2010:300–2, 539–40.

3. El Idrissi A, Messing J, Scalia J, et al. Prevention of epileptic seizures by taurine. *Adv Exp Med Biol* 2003;526:515–25.

4. Wynn SG, Marsden S. *Manual of natural veterinary medicine: science and tradition*. St. Louis (MO): Mosby; 2003:81, 323, 483, 500, 516, 589.

5. Stargrove M, Treasure J, McKee D. *Herb, nutrient, and drug interactions: clinical implications and therapeutic strategies*. St. Louis (MO): Mosby Elsevier; 2008:397, 553.

(L-TRYPTOPHAN, 5-HYDROXYTRYPTOPHAN, 5-HTP)

Background

Tryptophan is an essential amino acid that is used to synthesize niacin (vitamin B$_3$), the neurotransmitter serotonin (5-hydroxy-tryptamine), and the hormone melatonin (in the retina and pineal gland in the brain).[1] The richest sources of tryptophan are fish, meat (especially turkey), dairy, eggs, nuts, and wheat germ.[1] Most (98%) dietary tryptophan is metabolized into niacin.

The primary use of L-tryptophan is for depression and related disorders. The effectiveness of both L-tryptophan and 5-HTP as antidepressants is based on their ability to elevate serotonin levels.[1] In certain patients, supplementation with L-tryptophan is as effective as antidepressant drugs.[2]

L-tryptophan can enhance serotonin levels; however, 5-HTP is even more likely to elevate serotonin levels and cause "serotonin syndrome" (an autonomic dysfunction characterized by neuromuscular abnormalities and altered mental state), especially if combined with other medications that elevate serotonin levels.[1]

Eating a diet high in L-tryptophan (i.e., protein-based foods) does not significantly increase 5-HTP levels.[1] Synthetic L-tryptophan is manufactured by a fermentation process using glucose and 5-HTP is manufactured by extraction from the seeds of the African shrub *Griffonia simplicifolia*.[1]

Indications

Suggested Uses in Humans

- Acts as an antidepressant
- Helps patients with bipolar disorder, dementia, insomnia, migraine headaches, and various neuroses/psychoses

Suggested Uses in Dogs and Cats

- Acts as an antidepressant
- Helps minimize aggression (dogs)
- Curtails obsessive-compulsive disorder

Recommended Doses

In humans 0.5–12 g q 6–8 hr of L-tryptophan is recommended.[1] The daily dose of L-tryptophan should not exceed 1 g/45 kg body weight. Toxicity is more likely when the daily dose exceeds 7 g/68 kg/day. It may take up to 60 days before a full clinical response is seen.[1] The recommended dose of 5-HTP is 50–200 mg q 8–12 hr. An increased dose or a single dose of 5-HTP at night may be useful to enhance sleep.[1] In the author's experience, 10 mg/kg of L-tryptophan q 12 hr for dogs and 15–20 mg/kg q 12–24 hr for cats is recommended. Because of the potential for side effects and adverse reactions (described below) begin supplementation at the low end of the dose range.[1]

Side Effects

L-tryptophan and 5-HTP are generally considered safe if the contraindications and potential interactions with other medications or herbs are followed (described below).[2] In the late 1980s and early 1990s, the U.S. Food and Drug Administration (FDA) removed tryptophan from the market because of severe illness (i.e., eosinophilia-myalgia syndrome) and death resulting from intake of tryptophan. It was later determined that one manufacturer in Japan had used a new bacterial strain to synthesize the tryptophan and that this bacterium introduced toxic by-products that contaminated the supplement. Similar reactions from other supplements were identified, and it was determined that the contaminant rather than the tryptophan was responsible for these reactions.[1]

The main side effects typically reported by people taking L-tryptophan or 5-HTP include gastrointestinal symptoms (e.g., nausea, dry mouth), anxiety, dizziness, drowsiness, headache, and muscle pain. These symptoms tend to be observed at the higher end of the dose range.[1] People with liver disease may have a limited ability to metabolize 5-HTP.[1] People with autoimmune diseases may be more susceptible to adverse reactions when taking 5-HTP, and asthmatic patients may experience an exacerbation of their symptoms with administration of 5-HTP.[1]

Contraindications

L-tryptophan should be avoided in patients with cataracts, diabetes, psoriasis, bladder cancer, or achlorhydria (low or absent production of acid by the stomach). L-tryptophan may exacerbate rheumatoid arthritis.[1]

Interactions

L-tryptophan should be used cautiously (if at all) in patients taking medications that may elevate serotonin levels (e.g., selective serotonin reuptake inhibitors, SSRIs). Although in some cases tryptophan may be helpful when used with SSRIs (such as fluoxetine [Prozac]) to enhance the effectiveness of these medications in the treatment of depression, it should be used very cautiously to prevent serotonin syndrome.[1] Tryptophan should not be used with monoamine oxidase (MAO) inhibitors because of the possibility of increased risk of serotonin syndrome.[1] Tryptophan may also be useful when coadministered with tricyclic antidepressants (TCAs such as clomipramine, imipramine, and amitriptyline) to enhance the effectiveness of the TCAs in the treatment of depression, but should be used very cautiously to prevent serotonin syndrome.[1]

5-HTP should be avoided in patients taking any medications that may elevate serotonin levels (SSRIs, MAO inhibitors, TCAs) because of the high probability of inducing serotonin syndrome.[1] Although drugs that increase serotonin levels are less likely to be used in veterinary medicine than in human medicine, there are several MAO inhibitors that are commonly used in veterinary practice (e.g., amitraz, selegiline). Other drugs that might increase serotonin levels and/or possibly adversely interact with L-tryptophan and 5-HTP (e.g., clomipramine [Clomicalm], fluoxetine [Reconcile]) should be avoided. In contrast, allopurinol increases levels of tryptophan in the brain and could possibly be helpful when used with supplemental tryptophan for depression. More research is needed and close observation should be undertaken when using allopurinol with dietary tryptophan.[1] Combining lithium carbonate and tryptophan elevates levels of serotonin and cortisol (and may require dose reductions in lithium), but caution should be exercised to prevent serotonin syndrome and adverse alterations in cortisol level.[1] Large doses of tryptophan might interfere with the actions of the diazepam clorazepate.[1]

Tramadol has several mechanisms of action, including blocking serotonin reuptake in the brain. Simultaneous use of 5-HTP and L-tryptophan may increase the risk of side effects, including serotonin syndrome. Caution should be used with the coadministration of tramadol and 5-HTP or L-tryptophan.[1] Caution should also be used when combining 5-HTP with melatonin, SAMe, St. John's wort, or tryptophan because of the possibility of additive adverse effects.[1] L-tryptophan is considered a safer supplement than 5-HTP (i.e., less likely to cause significantly increased serotonin levels), and 5-HTP has a narrower therapeutic dose range and is much more likely to cause adverse reactions. Currently L-tryptophan is available only as a prescription medication, but 5-HTP is available as an over-the-counter supplement.[1]

References

1. Stargrove M, Treasure J, McKee D. *Herb, nutrient, and drug interactions: clinical implications and therapeutic strategies.* St Louis (MO): Mosby Elsevier; 2008:690–7, 706–17.

2. Pizzorno J, Murray M. *Textbook of natural medicine.* 3rd ed. St. Louis (MO): Churchill Livingstone; 2005:1436–8.

VALERIAN

(*VALERIANA OFFICINALIS*)

Background

Valerian, specifically the fresh or dried rhizomes, roots, and stolons, is a commonly used herb in people and pets as a mild sedative-hypnotic/anxiolytic.[1,2] The active ingredients in valerian include valepotriates, valerenic acid, amino acids, γ-aminobutyric acid (GABA), glutamine, lignans, flavonoids, alkaloids, and essential oils (sesquiterpenes).[3] The sedative effects of valerian are likely because of interactions with GABA receptors (i.e., GABA agonism).[4,5] Other effects may be associated with the melatonin receptors, serotonin receptors, H1 (histamine) receptors, and dopamine receptors.[6] Valerian improved the quality of sleep in insomniacs (comparable to benzodiazepine) but did not cause daytime sedation.[7] Valerian also has weak anticonvulsant properties.[8]

Valerian supplements typically have a characteristic strong odor. This herb can be administered alone, but in the author's experience, valerian is often combined with other sedative herbs, such as lemon balm, passionflower, and hops.

Indications

Suggested Uses in Humans
- Provides sedation
- Alleviates anxiety

Suggested Uses in Dogs and Cats
- Provides sedation
- Alleviates anxiety

Recommended Doses

In humans, recommended doses are 3–9 g of dried root or rhizome/day,[6] 2–6 mL of a 1:2 liquid extract/day, and 1–3 mL of a 1:1 tincture *q* 8 hr.[6] In dogs and cats, the dose of dried herb is 25–300 mg/kg/day (divided) and the tincture is dosed at 0.5–1.5 mL/10 kg/day (divided).[1]

Side Effects

Valerian is generally safe when used at recommended doses.

Contraindications

Valerian may potentiate the effects of central nervous system (CNS) depressants, and its use with similarly acting medications is generally contraindicated.[6]

Interactions

Combining valerian with other CNS depressant medications (e.g., benzodiazepines, anticonvulsants, anesthetics) should be avoided because of additive effects.[9] But valerian may be useful when attempting to reduce doses of medications such as benzodiazepines.[6] As with other CNS depressant herbs, it would be prudent to conclude that valerian should be withdrawn approximately 10 days before anesthesia.

References

1. Wynn SG, Fougère B. *Veterinary Herbal Medicine*. St. Louis (MO): Mosby Elsevier; 2007:657.

2. Broadfoot PJ, Palmquist RE, Jonston K, et al. *Integrating complementary medicine into veterinary practice*. Goldstein R, ed. Blackwell; 2008:649–707. Available at: www.mediafire.com/?2s13ctmvv7tyb2k. Accessed January 15, 2012.

3. Pizzorno J, Murray M. *Textbook of natural medicine*. 3rd ed. St. Louis (MO): Churchill Livingstone Elsevier; 2005:1371–3.

4. Wynn SG, Marsden S. *Manual of natural veterinary medicine: science and tradition*. St. Louis (MO): Mosby; 2003:51, 55, 86.

5. Schoen A, Wynn SG. *Complementary and alternative veterinary medicine: principles and practice*. St. Louis (MO): Mosby; 1998:333–4.

6. Stargrove M, Treasure J, McKee D. *Herb, nutrient, and drug interactions: clinical implications and therapeutic strategies*. St. Louis (MO): Mosby Elsevier; 2008:167–70.

7. Pizzorno J, Murray M, Joiner-Bey H. *The clinician's handbook of natural medicine*. 2nd ed. St. Louis (MO): Churchill Livingstone; 2008:431–2.

8. Fetrow CW, Avila J. *Professional's handbook of complementary and alternative medicines*. 3rd ed. Philadelphia (PA): Lippincott Williams & Wilkins; 2004:835–9.

9. Mills S, Bone K. *Principles and practice of phytotherapy: modern herbal medicine*. St. Louis (MS): Churchill Livingstone; 2000:581–8.

Background

"Vitamin A" is a generic term for a class of compounds that exhibit the same biologic activities as retinol—a yellow compound found in green and yellow vegetables, egg yolk, and fish liver oil that is essential for growth and vision. There are >600 carotenoids (highly colored plant pigments) that are considered "provitamin A nutrients." Examples include α-carotene, β-carotene, lutein, lycopene, cryptoxanthin, and zeaxanthin.[1] Mammals are able to convert carotenoids into retinol (vitamin A), except for cats, who cannot convert beta-carotene into vitamin A (they are lacking the necessary enzyme). Cats require preformed vitamin A in their diets to prevent deficiency.[2,3] Even if not converted to vitamin A in the body, carotenoids act as potent antioxidants.[3,4]

Retinoids (i.e., retinol, retinal, retinoic acid) occur only in animal products and are considered preformed vitamin A. Synthetic analogs of vitamin A include isotretinoin and acitretin, among others.[3] Vitamin A occurs in both a *cis* and a *trans* configuration (which refers to the "shape" of the molecule because of carbon-carbon double bonds). Both forms are biologically active, although vitamin A dietary supplements are typically the *trans* configuration.[1] Vitamin A is found in a number of dietary sources, including fish liver oil (especially cod liver oil), organ meats, egg yolk, and whole milk. Carotenoids are found in a variety of fruits and vegetables including yellow, red, and dark leafy green vegetables and yellow fruit.[1]

The liver stores 90% or more of the body's vitamin A content. In people, it can hold approximately 2 years' worth of vitamin A required by an adult.[1] Vitamin A is necessary for the body to fight infection, maintain immunity, and maintain integrity of the epithelium, and for bone growth, cellular differentiation, cellular proliferation, normal vision, and testicular and ovarian function.[1] Vitamin A is a cofactor in numerous biochemical reactions.[1] Vitamin A and the carotenoids are often indicated as part of the supportive care for patients with cancer.[6] The rationale for this recommendation is based on the fact that decreased intake of antioxidants is associated with increases in the adverse effects of chemotherapy and radiation therapy. Although this use of vitamin A and carotenoids remains controversial, integrative practitioners recommend using a mixture of antioxidants in chemotherapy and radiation therapy patients (please refer to Appendix 1 for a more in-depth discussion of this topic).

Vitamin A deficiencies are associated with impaired ability to mount an effective antibody response, decreased levels of helper T cells, and alterations in the mucosal linings of the respiratory and gastrointestinal tracts.[5]

Indications
Suggested Uses in Humans
- Functions as an antioxidant

Suggested Uses in Dogs and Cats
- Functions as an antioxidant

Recommended Doses
In humans, the recommended therapeutic dose of vitamin A is 25,000 international units (IU)/day. A maximum of 15,000 IU/day may be safer for older patients and those with liver disease, hypercholesterolemia, or diabetes (these patients are more likely to be predisposed to toxicity).[1] In dogs and cats, 625–7,500 IU/0.45 kg/day is recommended for the treatment of various cancers.[6] Alternatively, 5,000 IU/0.45 kg by injection *q* 3 weeks for various cancers (especially osteosarcoma) has been used successfully and safely by Dr. Steve Marsden (see reference list) as part of his vitamin therapy for cancer treatment.

Side Effects
Vitamin A and the carotenoids are generally considered safe when used as directed.

Contraindications
Large doses of vitamin A and most retinoids are contraindicated during pregnancy because of the possibility of embryo toxic effects; however, some studies have failed to detect an increase in birth defects in women receiving large doses of vitamin A during pregnancy.[1] Retinol supplementation is contraindicated in patients

with liver disease, and synthetic all *trans* β-carotene has been associated with an increased risk of lung cancer in smokers.[1]

Interactions

Oral neomycin impairs the absorption of vitamin A; therefore, supplemental vitamin A may be warranted in patients prescribed oral neomycin.[1] Similarly, patients being treated with antacids for gastric ulcers may benefit from vitamin A supplementation.[1] To prevent toxicity, patients using synthetic retinoids should not be administered vitamin A (particularly >10,000 IU/day in humans) without medical supervision.[1] Combining vitamin A with tetracycline antibiotics may increase the risk of benign intracranial hypertension (pseudotumor cerebri) in people.[1] Administering vitamin A with antibiotics may provide a synergistic effect.[1] Vitamin A may increase the potential for bleeding when combined with anticoagulant medications, and vitamin A is synergistic with chemotherapeutic cisplatin for head and neck cancers in humans.[1,7]

References

1. Stargrove M, Treasure J, McKee D. *Herb, nutrient, and drug interactions: clinical implications and therapeutic strategies.* St. Louis (MO): Mosby Elsevier; 2008:235–52.

2. Schoen A, Wynn SG. *Complementary and alternative veterinary medicine: principles and practice.* St. Louis (MO): Mosby; 1998:54, 60.

3. Hand M, Thatcher C, Remillard R, et al. *Small animal clinical nutrition.* 5th ed. Topeka (KS): Mark Morris Institute; 2010:84, 465.

4. Broadfoot PJ, Palmquist RE, Jonston K, et al. *Integrating complementary medicine into veterinary practice.* Goldstein R, ed. Blackwell; 2008:31–2, 137, 171, 721. Available at: www.mediafire.com/?2s13ctmvv7tyb2k. Accessed January 15, 2012.

5. Pizzorno J, Murray M. *Textbook of natural medicine.* 3rd ed. St. Louis (MO): Churchill Livingstone; 2005:771–3, 1382.

6. Wynn SG, Marsden S. *Manual of natural veterinary medicine: science and tradition.* St. Louis (MO): Mosby; 2003:121, 397.

7. Pizzorno J, Murray M, Joiner-Bey H. *The clinician's handbook of natural medicine.* 2nd ed. St. Louis (MO): Churchill Livingstone; 2008:131.

Background

Vitamin C is a water-soluble vitamin found primarily in fruits (especially citrus fruits) and vegetables[1] as well as organ meats. Most animals, including dogs and cats, can meet their dietary requirements for vitamin C from endogenous synthesis (i.e., from glucose via the glucuronic acid pathway) and do not have a specific dietary requirement for vitamin C. In times of illness, stress, and disease (such as cancer), an increased intake of vitamin C may be beneficial.[2] Vitamin C helps restore vitamin E's antioxidant activity,[3] is required for the synthesis of adrenal hormones and carnitine, and plays an essential role in the metabolism of a number of other compounds such as folic acid and tryptophan.[1] Vitamin C protects cholesterol from oxidative damage and lowers low-density lipoprotein (LDL, "bad" cholesterol) levels while increasing serum high-density lipoprotein (HDL, "good" cholesterol) levels.[1] Vitamin C works with lipoprotein-alpha to help reduce/dissolve atherosclerotic plaques.[1] Other important mechanisms of vitamin C relate to the immune system. Specifically, vitamin C increases lymphocyte production, macrophage activity, and antibody and interferon production.[3,4] In addition, vitamin C is important for the synthesis of collagen and elastin (in connective tissues) and inhibits hyaluronidase (the enzyme that breaks down hyaluronic acid). Thus, vitamin C is often included in joint supplements.[1] Additionally, vitamin C acts as a nitrate scavenger and may reduce nitrosamine-induced cancers,[1,2] and is necessary for the optimal activity of cytochrome mixed-function oxidases.[1]

It should be noted that high doses of vitamin C may cause copper depletion.[1] In contrast, vitamin C enhances the absorption of iron, but this benefit is likely to be of little clinical significance except in patients with iron overload or hemochromatosis.[1] When administered in concert with vitamin K_3, the combination is considered a pretreatment for radiation therapy and purportedly reduces tumor volume.[5] Vitamin C has also been used in patients with certain cancers.[6]

Indications

Suggested Uses in Humans
- Possesses antioxidant properties
- Supports cancer patients
- Helps resolve infections
- Improves symptoms of osteoarthritis

Suggested Uses in Dogs and Cats
- Possesses antioxidant properties
- Supports cancer patients
- Helps resolve infections
- Improves clinical signs of osteoarthritis

Recommended Doses

In humans, the dose of vitamin C is quite variable; 400 mg/day is thought to fully saturate plasma and cells.[1] In dogs and cats, similar doses are used.[6] In the author's experience vitamin C is administered at the "bowel tolerance" dose (i.e., the amount of vitamin C the patient can tolerate before loose stools or diarrhea is seen).

Caution must always be used when using megadoses of antioxidant vitamins and minerals in cancer patients (especially if isolated antioxidants are used). It is unknown what dose is considered safe, effective, or the "best." It is also unknown in what dose the vitamin or mineral acts as an antioxidant rather than as a pro-oxidant. More research is needed to answer these important questions.[1]

Side Effects

No major side effects secondary to vitamin C supplementation have been reported. That said, any antioxidant (vitamin or mineral) may, at high doses, act as a pro-oxidant rather than as an antioxidant.[7] The following mild side effects have been reported in people: gastrointestinal discomfort, flatulence, increased urination, skin rashes, and loose stools/diarrhea.[1,6] Chronic intake of high doses of vitamin C may result in a copper deficiency.[1] Many vitamin C supplements are synthesized from glucose by derivation from corn; patients with corn allergies may react to these supplements. Vitamin C supplements made from other sources (sago palm) would be safe to use in such patients.[1] Finally, supplemental vitamin C, especially at higher doses, may produce the following laboratory abnormalities: false negative results on fecal occult blood; false elevations of bilirubin, creatinine, aspartate aminotransferase (AST), and uric acid; false decreases in lactate dehydrogenase (LDH); and false negative or false positive results on urinary glucose tests (depending upon the methodology used).[7]

Contraindications

Supplemental vitamin C should not be administered to patients with cystinuria (a genetic condition causing cysteine stones to form in the urinary bladder) or hemosiderosis or hemochromatosis (iron overload disorders). In humans, doses ≥1,000 mg/day should not be used by patients with recurrent nephrolithiasis or oxalate cystic calculi (formation of stones in the urinary tract). Doses >4,000 mg/day should not be used by people with renal failure.[1] Similar precautions likely apply to dogs and cats as well. In people, it is recommended not to exceed 400 mg/day for at least 1 week prior to surgery because of the possibility of increased bleeding.[1]

Interactions

A number of interactions are worth mentioning here. Vitamin C has the potential to either increase or decrease serum levels of acetaminophen. Although acetaminophen is rarely used in veterinary medicine, extreme caution must be used if it is prescribed to patients also taking vitamin C supplements.[1] High-dose vitamin C may decrease endothelial damage in patients with hypertension.[1] High-dose intravenous vitamin C selectively kills cancer cells and reduces toxicity from chemotherapy medications.[1] On the downside, vitamin C may aggravate the cardiac toxicity of doxorubicin and other anthracyclines (chemotherapeutics) via mobilization of iron, which increases levels of iron-catalyzed free radicals.[1] Vitamin C is depleted during (prolonged) corticosteroid therapy, and supplementation might be beneficial.[1] Vitamin C can enhance the bioavailability of cyclosporine (an immunosuppressant) and may allow for decreased levels of cyclosporine as well as decreased side effects associated with cyclosporine.[1] Patients taking the diuretic furosemide might have a greater response to therapy when supplemented with vitamin C.[1] Patients taking statin drugs (to control blood pressure) may show improvement in lipid/cholesterol levels when they are coadministered with vitamin C.[1] Vitamin C may reduce the risk of *Helicobacter pylori* infection (which causes gastric ulcers); however, supplemental vitamin C should be avoided during therapy to treat *H. pylori,* as it may reduce therapeutic efficacy.[1] Vitamin C may have a synergistic effect if coadministered with nitroglycerin to help maintain/promote vasodilation.[1] Vitamin C may enhance the bioavailability and elevate blood levels of tetracycline (and potentially other antibiotics).[1] Vitamin C should not be administered with aluminum-containing antacids, as it can increase the absorption of aluminum.[1] Finally, patients prescribed anticonvulsants may benefit from supplemental vitamin C, as anticonvulsant medications may increase urinary excretion of vitamin C.[1]

References

1. Stargrove M, Treasure J, McKee D. *Herb, nutrient, and drug interactions: clinical implications and therapeutic strategies*. St. Louis (MO): Mosby Elsevier; 2008:356–98.

2. Hand M, Thatcher C, Remillard R, et al. *Small animal clinical nutrition*. 5th ed. Topeka (KS): Mark Morris Institute; 2010:94, 518, 895.

3. Wynn SG, Marsden S. *Manual of natural veterinary medicine: science and tradition*. St. Louis (MO): Mosby; 2003:137, 157.

4. Broadfoot PJ, Palmquist RE, Jonston K, et al. *Integrating complementary medicine into veterinary practice*. Goldstein R, ed. Blackwell; 2008:32–3, 132, 137. Available at: www.mediafire.com/?2s13ctmvv7tyb2k. Accessed January 15, 2012.

5. Pizzorno J, Murray M, Joiner-Bey H. *The clinician's handbook of natural medicine*. 2nd ed. St. Louis (MO): Churchill Livingstone; 2008:134.

6. Schoen A, Wynn SG. *Complementary and alternative veterinary medicine: principles and practice*. St. Louis (MO): Mosby; 1998:94, 101, 115–6, 118, 128.

7. Pizzorno J, Murray M. *Textbook of natural medicine*. 3rd ed. St. Louis (MO): Churchill Livingstone; 2005:567, 1491–5, 1764–75.

(CALCIFEROL, CALCITRIOL , 1,25-DIHYDROXYCHOLECALCIFEROL)

Background

Vitamin D is a fat-soluble vitamin and hormone. "Vitamin D" is a generic term for compounds that resemble, and have the activity of, calciferol, including vitamin D_2 (ergocalciferol), vitamin D_3 (cholecalciferol,) 1-α-hydroxycholecalciferol (alfacalcidol), 25-hydroxyvitamin D_3 (calcidiol, calcifediol), 1,25-dihydroxycholecaliferol (calcitriol), and dihydrotachysterol. Plant-based vitamin D_2 is called ergocalciferol, but is not as potent or bioavailable as cholecalciferol (vitamin D_3).[1]

Vitamin D either is available by absorption (from dietary sources) from the small intestine or is synthesized in the skin following exposure of cholesterol to ultraviolet B (UVB) radiation in sunlight.[1] Dogs and cats cannot rely on exposure to sunlight for vitamin D, as they have low activation of cholesterol in the skin by UVB light because of very low concentrations of cholesterol (7-dehydrocholesterol) in the skin.[2] Vitamin D_3 from dietary sources (e.g., cod liver oil, oily cold-water fish, butter, egg yolk), supplements, or following activation of cholesterol in the skin is subsequently converted in the liver to 25-hydroxycholecaliferol. In turn, 25-hydroxycholecaliferol is converted to the active form of vitamin D (i.e., calcitriol, 1,25-dihydroxycholecaliferol) in the kidneys.[2]

Current research indicates that many people are deficient in vitamin D. Vitamin D deficiency may be associated with an increased risk of diseases, including cancers, heart disease, hypertension, decreased immunity, multiple sclerosis, and diabetes.[1] Vitamin D deficiency can also result from Cushing's disease (hypoadrenocorticism), Crohn's disease/inflammatory bowel disease, hypothyroidism, kidney disease, liver disease, and anticonvulsant drug therapy.[1] Reduced exposure to sunlight, nonsupplemented vegetarian diets (vegetables are usually low in vitamin D), and the use of sunscreens that block ultraviolet B light rays are likely contributing factors. Because of the supplementation of processed pet foods, it is unlikely that either dogs or cats would become vitamin D deficient.[2] Vitamin D deficiency may be more of a problem with homemade diets that are not properly prepared.

Vitamin D is necessary for absorbing calcium and phosphorus from the intestine, regulating blood levels of calcium and phosphorus, facilitating mineral deposition into bone, maintaining adequate blood levels of insulin, assisting in metabolism of sugar, promoting healthy thyroid function (it may have a mechanism of action similar to that of thyroid hormone), assisting in regulation of cell growth and development, and promoting development, activity, and response of T cells against antigens and autoimmune disorders.[1] Naturopathic doctors are beginning to see the benefits of vitamin D in certain cancers, such as breast, prostate, lung, skin (melanoma), and bone. Vitamin D is also being used as part of an integrated therapeutic approach to the treatment of a variety of autoimmune diseases in people, especially type 1 diabetes, rheumatoid arthritis, and multiple sclerosis.[1]

Indications

Suggested Uses in Humans
- Benefits cancer patients
- Minimizes development of osteoporosis
- Ameliorates autoimmune diseases
- Helps patients with psoriasis (red, irritated skin) when used topically

Suggested Uses in Dogs and Cats
- Benefits cancer patients
- Minimizes development of osteoporosis

Recommended Doses

The current recommended dietary allowance (RDA) of vitamin D_3 for adults aged 19–50 years is 600 international units (IU)/day. Most naturopathic doctors recommend a minimum daily intake of 1,000–2,000 IU for healthy adults (and higher doses are used as part of integrative therapies for medical conditions). The exact dose is best determined by regularly monitoring plasma levels of vitamin D. Toxic vitamin D levels in adult humans are generally not reached until blood levels of at least >200 ng/mL are seen, which is unlikely with the usual recommended supplemental doses. Cod liver oil is often recommended as an excellent dietary source of vitamin D (5 mL [1 teaspoon] of cod liver oil provides approximately 1,200 IU [30 μg] of vitamin D_3).[2]

In humans, the dose of vitamin D for cancers and immune diseases is best determined by serial monitoring of plasma vitamin D levels. In general, doses from 2,000 IU to 10,000 IU/day are recommended.[3] In dogs and cats, the optimal dose of vitamin D for various cancers and immune diseases has not been determined. One dose that has been recommended (and used with success for the treatment of various cancers in dogs) is 750 IU/0.45 kg body weight administered *q* 3–4 weeks.[4]

Side Effects

Supplementation of vitamin D_3 is considered safe if excessive doses are not administered. Excessive doses from dietary sources and sunlight are considered highly unlikely. In people, it is believed that even oral vitamin D_3 doses >10,000–50,000 IU/day are unlikely to be associated with toxicity; however, adverse effects in people have been reported at concentrations ranging from 10,000 IU to 50,000 IU/day. Reported side effects in people include headache, kidney stones, and weight loss. Excess amounts of vitamin D may result in hypercalcemia and subsequent mineralization of blood vessels and body organs.[1]

In dogs and cats, vitamin D intoxication is most often the result of accidental or intentional poisoning through ingestion of cholecalciferol-containing rodenticides or human medications containing calcipotriol. A single oral toxic dose of cholecalciferol in a mature dog is approximately 80,000 IU/kg (2 mg/kg). A single oral toxic dose of calcipotriol in dogs is 50 μg/kg.[5,6]

Contraindications

People and pets with pre-existing conditions, including primary hyperparathyroidism, granulomatous disease, sarcoidosis, heart disease, arteriosclerosis, dehydration, primary renal failure, hypoadrenocorticism (i.e., Addison's disease), and lymphoma, are more susceptible to vitamin D intoxication. Supplementation with excessive amounts of vitamin D should be done cautiously (if at all) in these patients.[1] People (and possibly pets) with granulomatous diseases and certain types of lymphoma may quickly develop elevated levels of 1,25-dihydroxycholecaliferol because of autonomous conversion of its precursor, 25-hydroxyvitamin D. Human patients successfully treated (who achieve a complete response) for lymphoma may be cautiously supplemented with vitamin D_3 (however, regular monitoring of plasma levels of vitamin D is essential) because vitamin D deficiency is associated with increased risk of developing lymphoma and other cancers.[5,6]

Interactions

Anticonvulsant medications (such as phenobarbital) that induce cytochrome P450 and mixed-function oxidases (particularly CUP3A4) may result in decreased levels of vitamin D, leading to an increased risk of osteoporosis.[1] Cimetidine decreases the synthesis of vitamin D, resulting in decreased blood levels of vitamin D.[1] Long-term use of (oral) corticosteroids may cause osteoporosis because of reduced calcium absorption, decreased vitamin D availability, interference with vitamin D activation and metabolism, and decreased blood levels of vitamin D (inhaled and topical corticosteroid–containing medications are less likely to produce osteoporosis).[1] Thiazide diuretics may cause hypercalcemia by reducing calcium excretion and increasing blood levels of vitamin D.[1] Antituberculosis medications (e.g., isoniazid, rifampin, etc.) may cause vitamin D deficiency, especially when used for longer than 1 month.[1] Long-term use of neomycin can decrease absorption and/or increase elimination of vitamin D and other nutrients.[1] Calcium channel blockers, such as verapamil, can theoretically be antagonized by vitamin D supplementation, although this has not been reported clinically. Nonetheless, caution should be exercised when treating patients taking calcium channel blockers if vitamin D supplementation becomes necessary.[1]

The effects of doxorubicin chemotherapy may be enhanced when combined with supplemental vitamin D. In addition to promoting cell differentiation, supporting apoptosis (programmed cell death), and minimizing the chance of metastases and angiogenesis on its own, vitamin D may enhance the susceptibility of cancer cells (especially breast cancer cells in people) to doxorubicin-induced oxidative damage.[1] Because vitamin D increases calcium absorption and elevated blood calcium levels may potentiate the effects of cardiac glycosides, caution should be exercised in patients taking cardiac glycosides who may also benefit from vitamin D supplementation to ensure that cardiac glycoside toxicity/cardiac arrhythmias do not occur.[1] Finally, vitamin D deficiency may develop in patients taking ketoconazole for extended periods of time because of inhibition of the P450 enzymes that metabolize vitamin D, inhibition of 1,25-dihydroxycholecaliferol (calcitriol) synthesis, and decreased blood levels of calcitriol.[1]

References

1. Stargrove M, Treasure J, McKee D. *Herb, nutrient, and drug interactions: clinical implications and therapeutic strategies*. St. Louis (MO): Mosby Elsevier; 2008:399–421.

2. Hand M, Thatcher C, Remillard R, et al. *Small animal clinical nutrition*. 5th ed. Topeka (KS): Mark Morris Institute; 2010:84–6.

3. Life extension. Available at: http://www.lef.org/magazine/mag2006/mar2006_report_vitamind_01.htm?source=search&key=vitamin%20D%20cancer and http://www.lef.org/magazine/mag2010/sep2010_Michael-Holick-The-Pioneer-of-Vitamin-D-Research_01.htm?source=search&key=vitamin%20D%20cancer. Accessed February 21, 2012.

4. Wynn SG, Marsden S. *Manual of natural veterinary medicine: science and tradition*. St. Louis (MO): Mosby; 2003:398, 436, 452.

5. Peterson M, Talcott P. *Small animal toxicology*. Philadelphia (PA): WB Saunders; 2001:452–65.

6. Gfeller R, Messonnier S. *Handbook of small animal toxicology and poisonings*. 2nd ed. St. Louis (MO): Mosby; 2004:316–20, 431–3.

VITAMIN E

(ALPHA-TOCOPHEROL, α-TOCOPHEROL)

Background

Vitamin E and α-tocopherol, although used synonymously, are not synonymous. Vitamin E is technically a combination of four tocopherols (D-α-tocopherol, D-β-tocopherol, D-γ-tocopherol, and D-δ-tocopherol) and four tocotrienols (α-tocotrienol, D-β-tocotrienol, D-γ-tocotrienol, and D-δ-tocotrienol).[1] Vitamin E is synthesized only in plants. The richest sources are vegetable oils, followed by seeds and cereal grains. Tocopherol concentrations are highest in green leaves, whereas tocotrienols are found in the bran and germ parts of the plant.[2] There are two forms of α-tocopherol: D-α (natural) and DL-α (synthetic) forms.[1] As an antioxidant, vitamin E prevents lipid peroxidation, protects the stability of cell membranes, and protects fatty acids against oxidative damage.[1] Vitamin E reduces the formation of lipofuscin, which is an oxidized fat that contributes to aging.[1] Vitamin E is required to prevent oxidation of essential fatty acids (polyunsaturated fatty acids such as omega fatty acids).[1] Vitamin E inhibits platelet aggregation, affects the activity of immune and inflammatory cells, inhibits protein kinase C, and enhances vasodilation (dilation of blood vessels).[1] Vitamin E is necessary for normal neurological function and increases the metabolic activity of pregnane X receptors (thereby increasing detoxification of foreign substances/toxins).[1] Vitamin E also reduces the activity of cytochrome P450 enzymes.[1] There are reports that vitamin E acts as a pro-oxidant rather than an antioxidant when used in the synthetic form (DL-α-tocopherol) or when used as a sole antioxidant.[1]

Indications

Suggested Uses in Humans
- Acts as a potent antioxidant

Suggested Uses in Dogs and Cats
- Acts as a potent antioxidant

Recommended Doses

In humans, the recommended supplemental dose of vitamin E (i.e., α-tocopherol, D-α-tocopherol, or mixed tocopherols) is 400–2,500 IU/day.[1] In dogs and cats, recommended doses range from 400 IU to 2,000 IU/day or alternatively 20 IU/kg/day.[3]

Side Effects

Vitamin E is considered safe and is one of the least toxic vitamins. Most animals and people can tolerate high levels without side effects (although antagonism with other nutrients may occur at high doses). Rare side effects seen in people taking high doses of vitamin E for extended periods of time include fatigue, headache, bleeding, nausea, gastrointestinal distress, and muscular weakness.[1]

Contraindications

High doses of vitamin E in people (≥1,800 IU/day) may cause prolonged bleeding time and, theoretically, an increased risk of bleeding.[1] High doses of vitamin E should not be used in patients with hypertension or congestive heart failure (particularly if vitamin E is used as the sole antioxidant, as it may cause an increased risk of heart failure in patients taking angiotensin 1 converting enzyme [ACE] inhibitors).[1]

Interactions

Combining vitamin E with nonsteroidal anti-inflammatory drugs (NSAIDs such as acetylsalicylic acid [aspirin]) or anticoagulants may increase bleeding tendencies.[1] Topical vitamin E oil may reduce or prevent oral mucositis (inflammation of the lining of the gastrointestinal tract) associated with some forms of chemotherapy and radiation therapy.[1] Combining vitamin E with cisplatin may reduce the peripheral neuropathy that can occur with cisplatin therapy.[1] In addition, combining vitamin E with the immunomodulating drug cyclosporine may enhance the bioavailability of and decrease the clearance of cyclosporine, reduce side effects associated with cyclosporine, and allow lower drug dose levels.[1] Haloperidol may decrease vitamin E levels in the body. Combining vitamin E with haloperidol can prevent vitamin E deficiency (which occurs only rarely in dogs and cats).[1] Vitamin E may reduce the adverse effects of and enhance the therapeutic action of statin (blood pressure) medications.[1] Combining vitamin E with omeprazole may reduce mucosal damage because of erosive esophagitis.[1] Vitamin E may reduce ototoxicity and vestibular toxicity that can be seen with aminoglycoside medications (presumably because aminoglycosides induce free radical formation).[1]

Vitamin E administered with griseofulvin can elevate serum levels of griseofulvin, thus necessitating a reduced dose of griseofulvin.[1] Vitamin E may improve glucose tolerance in diabetics, possibly necessitating a reduced dose of insulin or oral hypoglycemic agents.[1] Combining vitamin E with synthetic retinoids can reduce dermatological side effects often seen with synthetic retinoids.[1] Anticonvulsant medications may lower serum levels of vitamin E; thus vitamin E supplementation could be considered for patients prescribed anticonvulsants.[1] Vitamin E, particularly if used as the sole antioxidant, may cause an increased risk of heart failure in patients taking ACE inhibitors.[1] Intake of high levels of polyunsaturated fatty acids/omega-3/omega-6 fatty acids can decrease vitamin E levels. For this reason, patients taking omega-3 fatty acid supplements should consider also supplementing with vitamin E; however, most fish oil supplements contain supplemental vitamin E (making additional supplementation unnecessary).[1]

References

1. Stargrove M, Treasure J, McKee D. *Herb, nutrient, and drug interactions: clinical implications and therapeutic strategies*. St. Louis (MO): Mosby Elsevier; 2008: 422–46.

2. Hand M, Thatcher C, Remillard R, et al. *Small animal clinical nutrition*. 5th ed. Topeka (KS): Mark Morris Institute; 2010:86–7, 466, 895.

3. Wynn SG, Marsden S. *Manual of natural veterinary medicine: science and tradition*. St. Louis (MO): Mosby; 2003:57, 80, 137–8, 370, 398.

APPENDIX 1

ADDITIONAL INFORMATION ON ANTIOXIDANTS

The term "antioxidant" refers to any substance (e.g., herb, nutritional supplement, vitamin, mineral, or endogenous chemical such as glutathione or superoxide dismutase) that prevents or minimizes oxidation. Oxidation is a reaction in which a molecule loses electrons and becomes unstable or "reactive." Molecules routinely become oxidized during cellular metabolism.[1] There are a number of antioxidants that can be used in clinical practice. A few of the more commonly used antioxidants are described throughout this book, including α-linoleic acid, and coenzyme Q_{10} (CoQ10).

Antioxidants are reportedly effective for a variety of medical problems in both people and animals. Common uses include autoimmune disorders, asthma, bronchitis, cognitive disorders, cardiac disease, renal disease, diabetes mellitus, degenerative myelopathy, osteoarthritis, atopic dermatitis, and seizures.[2,3]

One area of controversy worth noting is the use of antioxidants as part of the therapeutic regimen for patients with cancers.[2,4] Some doctors, especially oncologists and radiation therapists, are concerned that antioxidants might interfere with chemotherapy and/or radiation therapy. This is because of the fact that a few chemotherapy medications and all radiation therapies cause oxidization within the cancer cells that ultimately leads to the death of these cells (e.g., by lipid peroxidation and damaging DNA).[5] Additionally, the administration of only a few select (chemical) antioxidants (rather than using a balanced approach with multiple antioxidants), especially in patients consuming diets low in antioxidants, can cause some supplemental antioxidants to act as pro-oxidants rather than as antioxidants, which could contribute to worsening of the cancer. In fact, some studies using isolated antioxidants such as β-carotene (a colorful pigment in plants and precursor to vitamin A) have shown a worsening of certain cancers when these antioxidants are used along with chemotherapeutic agents or radiation therapy. These are the types of studies that doctors who are against the use of antioxidants in patients undergoing chemotherapy or radiation therapy cite when stating that antioxidants can be harmful when used in cancer patients. For example, one reported that using β-carotene increased lung cancer in men who also smoked.

However, several other types of cancer were reduced.[6] Additionally, synthetic β-carotene can reduce liver stores of other carotenoids, which are more important in cancer prevention than β-carotene (making synthetic β-carotene less desirable).[6] Studies that report an increase in cancer when antioxidants are used concomitantly with either chemotherapy or radiation should be closely scrutinized. These studies usually use an isolated, high dose of synthetic vitamins and may not be controlled for outside environmental factors such as smoking. Additionally, it should be kept in mind that cancer cells are not normal cells in their biochemistry, physiology, or metabolism. As such, cancer cells may react differently when exposed to various nutrients, including antioxidants, than normal cells. Because the interrelationship among antioxidants is complex, better results tend to occur when mixtures of antioxidants are used rather than when only one antioxidant is used.[6] For example, better results (i.e., clinical improvement) may occur when vitamins A, C, and E are used together rather than when only one of these antioxidant vitamins is used, because of the interactions among these vitamins.[3,6] Whenever possible, mixtures of antioxidants (especially natural antioxidants such as palm oil, which provides a mixture of tocopherols and tocotrienols rather than synthetic DL-α tocopherol, which is often referred to as "vitamin E") should be used to provide the best clinical improvement. In the author's opinion, many conventional oncologists do not properly address the nutritional needs of cancer patients and often recommend diets that tend to be antioxidant neutral or antioxidant deficient. These diets may promote cancer growth and metastasis rather than reduce or inhibit it.

When discussing cancer in general, it should be noted that each type of cancer has its own unique biology and can respond in its own individual and unique way to both conventional cancer therapies and natural cancer therapies. This makes it difficult to make blanket or general recommendations for using antioxidants in specific cancers without well-designed clinical studies. For example, it may be that melanoma is best treated with a certain mixture of antioxidants whereas squamous cell carcinoma might be better treated with a different group of antioxidants. Much more research is needed to fully elucidate the effects of various nutrients on each type of cancer.

Veterinarians are often forced to apply *in vitro* results to patients or to extrapolate recommendations from *in vivo* studies in people. Alas, there are inherent difficulties with this approach. Once again, further research in each species of patient using a variety of antioxidants for each type of cancer will provide more information to better guide veterinarians in selecting the most appropriate supplement(s) to use in patients.

Despite all of these concerns, doctors practicing integrative medicine often employ antioxidants as part of their integrative therapy for treating a patient with cancer. The rationale behind antioxidant usage as part of a balanced therapeutic approach to the patient with cancer is as follows:

1. Chemotherapy and/or radiation therapy, because of its oxidizing effect on cells through the generation of free radicals, often causes decreased levels of antioxidants within the cells and/or plasma.

2. Antioxidants induce cell differentiation and growth inhibition by blocking damage from free radicals (protecting healthy cells) and inhibiting the enzyme protein kinase C activity.[1] In turn, tumor cell division and proliferation are inhibited, the expression of cancer-promoting genes is inhibited, transforming growth factor β and p21 genes are induced, and the growth-inhibiting effects of radiation therapy and chemotherapy are enhanced.

3. Certain conventional medicines (such as CoQ10) are often employed in concert with chemotherapy because of their antioxidant effects that limit tissue damage caused by the oxidizing effects of the chemotherapy medication. These antioxidant medications in no way interfere with the cancer cell–killing ability of chemotherapy.

To date, there are no credible reports or controlled clinical studies to support the fear that antioxidant usage interferes with the cancer-killing effects of chemotherapy or radiation therapy. On the contrary, the use of antioxidants during conventional cancer therapies will more likely be helpful (or at worst exhibit negligible efficacy) than harmful. Supplement usage during chemotherapy and/or radiation therapy, especially supplement therapy with antioxidants, often increases the efficacy of the conventional therapy while minimizing side effects from the conventional therapy.[2] Theoretically, antioxidant usage during chemotherapy with certain chemotherapeutic agents might actually allow for a reduced dose of the chemotherapeutic agent without sacrificing efficacy. Oxidative damage occurs to all cells (not just cancer cells) during chemotherapy or radiation therapy. Because excessive oxidation is a known cause of cancer, the use of antioxidants is likely to protect noncancerous cells from damage.

At this time, research plus clinical experience tends to support the use of a balanced antioxidant regimen when combined with a proper diet for patients treated with chemotherapy and/or radiation therapy, regardless of the type of cancer present. The practitioner is encouraged to constantly monitor the cancer patient to assess efficacy of the conventional therapies (as well as any natural therapies) and to note any side effects that may arise during integrative cancer therapy.

References

1. Broadfoot PJ, Palmquist RE, Jonston K, et al. *Integrating complementary medicine into veterinary practice.* Goldstein R, ed. Blackwell; 2008:706–7, 721–2. Available at: www.mediafire.com/?2s13ctmvv7tyb2k. Accessed January 15, 2012.

2. Wynn SG, Marsden S. *Manual of natural veterinary medicine: science and tradition.* St. Louis (MO): Mosby; 2003:51, 57, 271, 420, 532.

3. Schoen A, Wynn SG. *Complementary and alternative veterinary medicine: principles and practice.* St. Louis (MO): Mosby; 1998:115–9.

4. Pizzorno J, Murray M, Joiner-Bey H. *The clinician's handbook of natural medicine.* 2nd ed. St. Louis (MO): Churchill Livingstone; 2008:134–5.

5. Stargrove M, Treasure J, McKee D. *Herb, nutrient, and drug interactions: clinical implications and therapeutic strategies.* St. Louis (MO): Mosby Elsevier; 2008:179–80, 242–3.

6. Blaylock R. *Natural strategies for cancer patients.* New York: Kensington Publishing Corp.; 2003:132–3, 156–9.

APPENDIX 2

LIST OF SUPPLEMENTS THAT MAY AFFECT BLOOD COAGULATION

- Coenzyme Q_{10}
- Dehydroepiandrosterone (DHEA)
- Fish Oil (Linseed oil, *Linum usitatissimum*)
- Garlic (*Allium sativum*)
- Ginkgo (*Ginko biloba*)
- Green Tea (*Camellia sinensis*)
- Hawthorn (*Crataegus laevigata, C. monogyna, C. oxyacantha*)
- Kava (*Piper methysticum*)
- S-adenosylmethionine (SAMe)
- St. John's Wort (*Hypericum perforatum*)
- Super Green Foods: Spirulina/Blue-Green Algae (*Spirulina platensis, S. maxima*)
- Vitamin A
- Vitamin C
- Vitamin E

APPENDIX 3

LIST OF SUPPLEMENTS THAT MAY INTERACT WITH ANESTHETICS, SEDATIVES, AND ANTIDEPRESSANTS

- Dehydroepiandrosterone (DHEA)
- Ginkgo (*Ginko biloba*)
- Kava (*Piper methysticum*)
- S-adenosylmethionine (SAMe)
- St. John's Wort (*Hypericum perforatum*)
- Valerian (*Valeriana officinalis*)

APPENDIX 4

LIST OF SUPPLEMENTS THAT MAY REDUCE SIDE EFFECTS FROM AND/OR ENHANCE CYTOTOXICITY OF CHEMOTHERAPY AND RADIATION THERAPY

- Carnitine (L-carnitine)
- Chondroitin (may also be contraindicated depending on the type of neoplasm)
- Coenzyme Q_{10}
- Fish Oil (Linseed oil, *Linum usitatissimum*)
- Garlic (*Allium sativum*)
- Ginkgo (*Ginko biloba*)
- Green Tea (*Camellia sinensis*)
- Melatonin (N-acetyl-5-methoxytryptophan)
- Silymarin/Milk Thistle (*Silybum marianum*)

LIST OF REFERENCES

Agency for Toxic Substances and Disease Registry (ATSDR). ToxFAQs for silver. Available at: http://www.atsdr.cdc.gov/toxfaqs/tf.asp?id=538&tid=97. Accessed January 9, 2012.

Alejandro A, Stamenkovic I, Meinick M, et al. CD44 is the principal cell surface receptor for hyaluronate. *Cell* 1990;61:1303–13.

Baker NF, Farver TB. Failure of brewer's yeast as a repellant to fleas on dogs. *J Am Vet Med Assoc* 1983;183(2):212–4.

Blaylock R. *Natural strategies for cancer patients.* New York: Kensington Publishing Corp.; 2003:132–3, 156–9.

Broadfoot PJ, Palmquist RE, Jonston K, et al. *Integrating complementary medicine into veterinary practice.* Goldstein R, ed. Blackwell; 2008:541. Available at: www.mediafire.com/?2s13ctmvv7tyb2k. Accessed January 15, 2012.

Brown MB, Jones SA. Hyaluronic acid: a unique topical vehicle for the localized delivery of drugs to the skin. *J Eur Acad Dermatol Venereol* 2005;19(3):308–18.

ConsumerLab.com. Product review: *Probiotics for adults, children and pets.* Available at: https://www.consumerlab.com/reviews/Probiotic_Supplements _Lactobacillus_acidophilus_Bifidobacterium/probiotics/. Accessed February 21, 2012.

Cooper C, Brown K, Meletis C, et al. Inflammation and hyaluronic acid. *Altern Compl Ther* 2008;14(2):78–84.

Dharmananda S. *Amino acid supplements 1: glutamine. With Reference to the Related Compound Glutamate.* Available at: http://www.itmonline.org/arts /glutamine.htm. Accessed March 13, 2012.

El Idrissi A, Messing J, Scalia J, et al. Prevention of epileptic seizures by taurine. *Adv Exp Med Biol* 2003;526:515–25.

Fetrow CW, Avila J. *Professional's handbook of complementary & alternative medicines.* 3rd ed. Philadelphia (PA): Lippincott Williams & Wilkins; 2004.

Fung MC, Bowen DL. Silver products for medical indications: risk-benefit assessment. *J Toxicol Clin Toxicol* 1996;34(1):119–26.

Gfeller R, Messonnier S. *Handbook of small animal toxicology and poisonings.* 2nd ed. St. Louis (MO): Mosby; 2004:316–20, 431–3.

Graeser AC, Giller K, Wiegand H, et al. Synergistic chondroprotective effect of alpha-tocopherol, ascorbic acid, and selenium as well as glucosamine and chondroitin on oxidant induced cell death and inhibition of matrix metalloproteinase-3—studies in cultured chondrocytes. *Molecules* 2009; 15:27–39.

Gulbranson SH, Hud JA, Hansen RC. Argyria following the use of dietary supplements containing colloidal silver protein. *Cutis* 2000;66(5):373–4.

Habib MAB, Parvin M, Huntington TC, et al. A review on culture, production and use of Spirulina as food for humans and feeds for domestic animals and fish. FAO Fisheries and Aquaculture Circular No. 1034. 2008. Available at: ftp://ftp.fao.org/docrep/fao/011/i0424e/i0424e00.pdf. Accessed March 12, 2012.

Hand M, Thatcher C, Remillard R, et al. *Small animal clinical nutrition*. 5th ed. Topeka (KS): Mark Morris Institute; 2010.

Hixson O. Acute intragastric toxicity (LD-50). Dimethyl sulfone (methyl-sulfonylmethane, MSM). Laboratory of Vitamin Technology, Inc., Chicago, IL, August 21, 1958.

Kalman DS, Heimer M, Valdeon A, et al. Effect of a natural extract of chicken combs with a high content of hyaluronic acid (Hyal-Joint®) on pain relief and quality of life in subjects with knee osteoarthritis: a pilot randomized double-blind placebo-controlled trial. *Nutr J* 2008;7:3.

Kendall R. *Building wellness with DMG*. Topanga (CA): Freedom Press; 2003.

Kim LS, Axelrod LJ, Howard P, et al. Efficacy of methylsulfonylmethane (MSM) in osteoarthritis pain of the knee: a pilot clinical trial. *Osteoarthritis Cartilage* 2006 14(3):286–94.

Lee KW, Yamato O, Tajima M, et al. Hematologic changes associated with the appearance of eccentrocytes after intragastric administration of garlic extract to dogs. *Am J Vet Res* 2000;61(11):1446–50.

Li CJ, Zhang QM, Li MZ, et al. Attenuation of myocardial apoptosis by alpha-lipoic acid through suppression of mitochondrial oxidative stress to reduce diabetic cardiomyopathy. *Chin Med J* [Engl] 2009;122(21):2580–6.

Loftin EG, Herold LV. Therapy and outcome of suspected alpha lipoic acid toxicity in two dogs. *J Vet Emerg Crit Care* [San Antonio] 2009;19(5):501–6.

Mayo Clinic. Consumer health. Question: colloidal silver: is it safe or effective? Available at: www.mayoclinic.com/health/colloidal-silver/AN01682. Accessed January 9, 2012.

McNamara PS, Barr SC, Erb HN. Hematologic, hemostatic, and biochemical effects in dogs receiving an oral chondroprotective agent for thirty days. *Am J Vet Res* 1996;57:1390–4.

Memorial Sloan-Kettering Cancer Center. Transfer factor. About herbs, botanicals & other products. Available at: http://www.mskcc.org/cancer-care/herb/transfer-factor. Accessed March 12, 2012.

Messonnier SP. *The natural health bible for dogs & cats: your A-Z guide to over 200 herbs, vitamins, and supplements*. New York: Three Rivers Press; 2001.

Mills S, Bone K. *Principles and practice of phytotherapy: modern herbal medicine*. St. Louis (MO): Churchill Livingstone; 2000.

National Institutes of Health. National Center for Complementary and Alternative Medicine (NCCAM). Backgrounder: colloidal silver products. Available at: http://nccam.nih.gov/health/silver/. Accessed January 9, 2012.

National Institutes of Health. National Center for Complementary and Alternative Medicine. What is complementary and alternative medicine? Available at: http://nccam.nih.gov/health/whatiscam/. Accessed January 15, 2012.

Olczyk P, Komosińska-Vassev K, Winsz-Szczotka K, et al. [Hyaluronan: structure, metabolism, functions, and role in wound healing]. *Postepy Hig Med Dosw (Online).* 2008;62:651–9 [in Polish].

Packaged Facts. Pet supplements and nutraceutical treats in the U.S. 3rd ed. February 2011. Available at: https://www.packagedfacts.com/Pet-Supplements -Nutraceutical-2588715/. Accessed January 15, 2012.

Peterson M, Talcott P. *Small animal toxicology.* Philadelphia (PA): WB Saunders; 2001:452–65.

Pizzorno J, Murray M. *Textbook of natural medicine.* 3rd ed. St. Louis (MO): Churchill Livingstone; 2006.

Pizzorno J, Murray M, Joiner-Bey H. *The clinician's handbook of natural medicine.* 2nd ed. St. Louis (MO): Churchill Livingstone; 2008:559.

Sawitzke AD, Shi H, Finco MF, et al. Clinical efficacy and safety over two years use of glucosamine, chondroitin sulfate, their combination, celecoxib or placebo taken to treat osteoarthritis of the knee: a GAIT report. *Ann Rheum Dis* 2010;69:1459–64. Available at: http://www.ncbi.nlm.nih.gov/pmc/articles /PMC3086604/pdf/nihms267850.pdf. Accessed February 19, 2010.

Schoen AM, Wynn SG. *Complementary and alternative veterinary medicine: principles and practice.* St. Louis (MO): Mosby; 1998.

Scott D, Miller W, Griffin C. *Muller and Kirk's small animal dermatology.* 6th ed. Philadelphia (PA): WB Saunders Company; 2001.

Simon RR, Marks V, Leeds AR, et al. A comprehensive review of oral glucosamine use and effects on glucose metabolism in normal and diabetic individuals. *Diabetes Metab Res Rev* 2011;27(1):14–27. Available at: http://www.ncbi.nlm.nih.gov/pmc /articles/PMC3042150/pdf/dmrr0027-0014.pdf. Accessed February 20, 2012.

Stargrove M, Treasure J, McKee D. *Herb, nutrient, and drug interactions: clinical implications and therapeutic strategies.* St. Louis (MO): Mosby Elsevier; 2008.

Strauss EJ, Hart JA, Miller MD, et al. Hyaluronic acid viscosupplementation and osteoarthritis: current uses and future directions. *Am J Sports Med* 2009;37(8):1636–44.

Suksomboon N, Poolsup N, Boobkaew S, et al. Meta-analysis of the effect of herbal supplement on glycemic control in type 2 diabetes. *J Ethnopharmacol* 2011;137(3):1328–33.

Teng YH, Tan PH, Chia SJ, et al. Increased expression of non-sulfated chondroitin correlates with adverse clinicopathological parameters in prostate cancer. *Mod Pathol* 2008;21(7):893–901.

U.S. Department of Health and Human Services. United States Food and Drug Administration. Overview of dietary supplements. Available at: http://www .fda.gov/Food/DietarySupplements/ConsumerInformation/ucm110417 .htm#what. Accessed January 15, 2012.

U.S. Food and Drug Administration. Colloidal silver not approved. Available at: http://www.fda.gov/AnimalVeterinary/NewsEvents/CVMUpdates/ucm127976 .htm. Accessed February 19, 2012.

Usha PR, Naidu MU. Randomised, double-blind, parallel, placebo-controlled study of oral glucosamine, methylsulfonylmethane, and their combination in osteoarthritis. *Clin Drug Investig* 2004;24(6):353–63.

Vázquez JA, Montemayor MI, Fraguas J, et al. Hyaluronic acid production by *Streptococcus zooepidemicus* in marine by-products media from mussel processing wastewaters and tuna peptone viscera. *Microb Cell Fact* 2010;9:46.

Wander RC, Hall JA, Gradin JL, et al. The ratio of dietary (n-6) to (n-3) fatty acids influences immune system function, eicosanoid metabolism, lipid peroxidation and vitamin E status in aged dogs. *J Nutr* 1997;127(6):1198–205.

Weese JS, Arroyo L. Bacteriological evaluation of dog and cat diets that claim to contain probiotics. Can Vet J 2003;44(3):212–5. Available at: http://www .ncbi.nlm.nih.gov/pmc/articles/PMC340078/pdf/20030300s00016p212.pdf. Accessed February 20, 2012.

Weindl G, Schaller M, Schäfer-Korting M, et al. Hyaluronic acid in the treatment and prevention of skin diseases: molecular biological, pharmaceutical and clinical aspects. *Skin Pharmacol Physiol* 2004;17(5):207–13.

White JM, Powell AM, Brady K, et al. Severe generalized argyria secondary to ingestion of colloidal silver protein. *Clin Exp Dermatol* 2003;28(3):254–6.

Wynn SG, Fougère B. *Veterinary herbal medicine*. St. Louis (MO): Elsevier; 2007.

Wynn SG, Marsden S. *Manual of natural veterinary medicine: science and tradition*. St. Louis (MO): Mosby; 2002.

FURTHER READING

Alejandro A, Stamenkovic I, Meinick M, et al. CD44 is the principal cell surface receptor for hyaluronate. *Cell* 1990;61(7):1303–13.

Andrews GP, Laverty TP, Jones DS. Mucoadhesive polymeric platforms for controlled drug delivery. *Eur J Pharmaceutics and Biopharmaceutics* 2009;71(3):505–18.

Arthur J, O'Brien ME, Subak-Sharpe G, eds. *Nutraceuticals: the complete encyclopedia of supplements, herbs, vitamins, and healing foods.* New York: Perigee; 2001.

Bosworth TR, Scott JE. A specific fluorometric assay for hexosamines in glycosaminoglycans, based on deaminative cleavage with nitrous acid. *Anal Biochem* 1994;223(2);266–73.

Bratman S, Kroll D. *The natural health bible:your A-Z guide to over 200 herbs, vitamins, and supplements,* Prima; 1999.

Cooper R, Kronenberg F, eds. *Botanical medicine: from bench to bedside.* New Rochelle (NY): Mary Ann Liebert, Inc. Publishers; 2009.

Fundukian L, ed. *The Gale encyclopedia of alternative medicine.* 3rd ed. Gale Cengage; 2008.

Hill AS, Werner JA, Rogers QR, et al. Lipoic acid is 10 times more toxic in cats than reported in humans, dogs or rats. *J Anim Physiol Anim Nutr* [Berl] 2004;88(3–4):150–6.

Ialenti A, Di Rosa M. Hyaluronic acid modulates acute and chronic inflammation. *Agents Actions* 1994:43(1–2):44–7.

Kawcak CE, Frisbie DD, Trotter GW, et al. Effects of intravenous administration of sodium hyaluronate on carpal joints in exercising horses after arthroscopic surgery and osteochondral fragmentation. *Am J Vet Res* 1997;58(10):1132–40.

Lininger S, Gaby A, Sutin S, et al. *The natural pharmacy: complete home reference to natural medicine.* New York: Three Rivers Press; 1999.

Medleau L, Hnilica K. *Small animal dermatology: a color atlas and therapeutic guide.* St. Louis (MO): Elsevier; 2006.

Meletis C, Zabriskie N, Rountree R. *Clinical natural medicine handbook.* New Rochelle (NY): Mary Ann Liebert, Inc. Publishers; 2008.

Schenck P. *Home-prepared dog and cat diets.* 2nd ed. Ames (IA): Wiley-Blackwell; 2010.

Schwartz S. *Psychoactive herbs in veterinary behavior medicine.* Ames (IA): Blackwell Publishing; 2005.

Sobocinski PZ, Canterbury WJ, Jurgens KH. Improved continuous-flow method for determination of total serum hexosamines. *Clin Chem* 1976;22(8):1394–6.

Tilford G, Wulff-Tilford M. *Herbs for pets: the natural way to enhance your pet's life*. 2nd ed. Irvine (CA): BowTie Press; 2009.

Washington K, Gottfried MR, Telen MJ. Expression of the cell adhesion molecule CD44 in gastric adenocarcinomas. *Hum Pathol* 1994;25(10):1043–9.

Wright KE, Maurer SG, DiCesare PE. Viscosupplementation for osteoarthritis. *Am J Orthop* 2000;29(2):18–89.

Wynn SG. *Emerging therapies: using herbs and nutraceutical supplements for small animals*. Lakewood (CO): AAHA Press; 1999.

Yarnell E, Abascal K, Rountree R. *Clinical botanical medicine*. 2nd ed. New Rochelle (NY): Mary Ann Liebert, Inc. Publishers; 2009.

ABOUT THE AUTHOR

Shawn Messonnier, DVM, graduated from Texas A&M College of Veterinary Medicine in 1987. He is an award-winning author of 30 books including *The Natural Health Bible for Dogs & Cats: Your A-Z Guide to over 200 Conditions, Herbs, Vitamins, and Supplements* (Three Rivers Press), *The Natural Vet's Guide to Preventing and Treating Cancer in Dogs* (New World Library), *The Natural Vet's Guide to Preventing and Treating Arthritis in Dogs and Cats* (New World Library), *8 Weeks to a Healthy Dog* (Rodale), *The Allergy Solution for Dogs: Natural and Conventional Therapies to Ease Discomfort and Enhance Your Dog's Quality of Life* (Three Rivers Press), and *Unexpected Miracles: Hope and Holistic Healing for Pets* (Forge Books). Messonnier is also a radio show host of *Dr. Shawn–The Natural Vet*, on Martha Stewart Living Radio (on Sirius/XM radio). His website, www.petcarenaturally.com, is consistently ranked number one on search engines. He is a sought-after speaker on the topic of natural pet care and veterinary marketing and entertains audiences with his award-winning magic/mentalist act.